Uprooting and Surviving

PRIORITY ISSUES IN MENTAL HEALTH

*A book series published under the auspices of
The World Federation for Mental Health*

EDITORIAL COMMITTEE

Chairman: MORTON BEISER *(Canada)*
G. MORRIS CARSTAIRS *(U.S.A.)*
T. E. D. VAN DER GRINTEN *(The Netherlands)*
SUSAN BUTT *(Canada)*
RICHARD C. NANN *(Canada)*
JEAN-LOUIS ARMAND-LAROCHE *(France)*
EUGENE B. BRODY *(U.S.A.)*

VOLUME 2

Uprooting and Surviving

Adaptation and Resettlement
of Migrant Families and Children

Edited by

RICHARD C. NANN, D. S. W.

School of Social Work, University of British Columbia

D. REIDEL PUBLISHING COMPANY

DORDRECHT : HOLLAND / BOSTON : U.S.A.
LONDON : ENGLAND

Library of Congress Cataloging in Publication Data

Main entry under title:

Uprooting and surviving.

(Priority issues in mental health ; v. 2)
Includes index.
  1.   Emigration and immigration—Psychological aspects—Addresses, essays, lectures. 2. Assimilation (Sociology)—Addresses, essays, lectures, I. Nann, Richard C. II. Series. [DNLM: 1. Refugees—Psychology—Congresses. 2. Emigration and immigration—Congresses. 3. Transients and migrants—Psychology—Congresses. 4. Mental health —Congresses. W1 PR524R / WA 305 U68 1977–79]
JV6127.U65   304.8   81–15358
ISBN-13: 978-94-009-7736-5   e-ISBN-13:978-94-009-7734-1
DOI: 10.1007/978-94-009-7734-1

Published by D. Reidel Publishing Company,
P.O. Box 17, 3300 AA Dordrecht, Holland.

Sold and distributed in the U.S.A. and Canada
by Kluwer Boston Inc.
190 Old Derby Street, Hingham, MA 02043, U.S.A.

In all other countries, sold and distributed
by Kluwer Academic Publishers Group,
P.O. Box 322, 3300 AH Dordrecht, Holland

D. Reidel Publishing Company is a member of the Kluwer Group

All Rights Reserved
Copyright © 1982 by D. Reidel Publishing Company, Dordrecht, Holland
Softcover reprint of the hardcover 1st edition 1982
No part of the material protected by this copyright notice may be reproduced or
utilized in any form or by any means, electronic or mechanical,
including photocopying, recording or by any information storage and
retrieval system, without written permission from the copyright owner

FOREWORD

The publication of this volume is significant in three respects. First, it represents a major concern of the international mental health movement in its effort to gain deeper understanding of migration and its mental health implications in our increasingly mobile modern societies. Second, it epitomizes continuous international cooperation of colleagues dedicated to the cause of tackling this important mental health problem. Third, it stands as another milestone in the growth of the World Federation for Mental Health through its biennial world congresses.

I sincerely hope that the empirical observations of real-life events contained in this volume will stimulate others to add their own experiences and perspectives on these topics at future congresses. It is also hoped that certain models of problem solving reported by the collaborators of this book may find wider application and that the results will be communicated to others. It is through such ensuing developments that the World Federation for Mental Health wishes to, and can, fulfill its roles of advocacy and international communication in promoting international mental health.

My gratitude goes to Richard Nann and his colleagues for having made this timely contribution available.

TSUNG-YI LIN, M.D., F.R.C.P. (C)
Honorary President, WFMH

TABLE OF CONTENTS

TSUNG-YI LIN / Foreword	v
RICHARD C. NANN / Preface	xi
MARIA PFISTER-AMMENDE / Prologue	xv
RICHARD C. NANN / Uprooting and Surviving – An Overview	1
KEH-MING LIN, MINORU MASUDA, and LAURIE TAZUMA / Problems of Vietnamese Refugees in the United States	11
MINORU MASUDA, KEH-MING LIN, and LAURIE TAZUMA / Life Changes among the Vietnamese Refugees	25
NORMAN V. LOURIE / Innovative Mental Health Services for Indo-Chinese Refugees in the United States	35
JOE YAMAMOTO / Beginning an Asian/Pacific Mental Health Clinic	41
A. L. Th. VERDONK / The Children of Immigrants in the Netherlands: Social Position and Implied Risks for Mental Health	49
BRITT-INGRID STOCKFELT-HOATSON / Education and Socialisation of Migrants' Children in Sweden with Special Reference to Bilingualism and Biculturalism	71
MARY ASHWORTH / The Cultural Adjustment of Immigrant Children in English Canada	77
BEVERLY NANN / Settlement Programs for Immigrant Women and Families	85
BEN CHUD / The Threshold Model: A Conceptual Framework for Understanding and Assisting Children of Immigrants	95
GEORGE V. COELHO / The Foreign Student's Sojourn as a High Risk Situation: The "Culture-Shock" Phenomenon Re-examined	101
AKIRA HOSHINO / An Elaboration of the "Culture-Shock" Phenomenon: Adjustment Problems of Japanese Youth Returning from Overseas	109
ALI NAHIT BABAOGLU / Some Social and Psychiatric Aspects of Uprooting among Turkish Immigrant Workers in West Germany	111
MORTON BEISER / Migration in a Developing Country: Risk and Opportunity	119
K. Y. MAK and SYLVIA C. L. CHEN / Mental Health of Mainland Chinese in Hong Kong	147
RICHARD C. NANN and LILIAN TO / Experiences of Chinese Immigrants in Canada: (A) Building an Indigenous Support System	155

K. C. LI and HEATHER LUK / Experiences of Chinese Immigrants in
    Canada: (B) Mental Health Services 165
MEI-CHEN LIN / Experiences of Chinese Immigrants in Canada: (C)
    Patterns of Help-Seeking and Socio-Cultural Determinants 175

LIST OF CONTRIBUTORS 187

INDEX OF NAMES 189

INDEX OF SUBJECTS 193

*This book is dedicated to Sander and Andrea,
two beautiful products of migrant families.*

PREFACE

To many people in the world, mobility is equated with opportunity, and the freedom to move is cherished as a fundamental right. On the other hand, the act of migrating and the pulling up of roots is neither opportune nor a matter of choice to the millions of persons, such as political refugees, who have become displaced from their homes by events beyond their control.

The papers in this volume concern families and children who are uprooted, whether by choice or by force of circumstances. This theme is hardly a new one in world history. Indeed, it would be difficult to find an era when some movement of people did not occur, and it might even be said that mobility seems to be a timeless part of the human condition. But in spite of the eons of human experience, and notwithstanding the considerable research given to the subject in recent years, large gaps remain in our knowledge about the phenomenon of migration and the adaptive patterns of migrants as they resettle in a new environment. At the same time, the need for a better understanding of these matters is more urgent than ever today as various international, national, and local agencies and organizations grapple with a multitude of problems and challenges arising from the movement and relocation of refugees and other migrant populations.

This volume offers some new perspectives on the nature and effects of uprooting and on the complex processes involved in resettlement. Its contents are wide-ranging and include reports from many different regions of the world. In most of the instances, the experiences described are still going on, as indicated in papers concerning such topics as, for example: the adaptation of Southeast-Asian refugees in the United States; the experience of immigrant populations in North America, Europe, and Asia; the changing mobility and life styles of West Africans as a consequence of industrialization and modernization; the status of foreign workers in Europe; and the special problems of youth trying to fit back into their home societies after several years of absence due to reasons such as studying abroad.

Although these topics are, as already noted, very wide-ranging and diverse, some common themes may be discerned threading through the papers. A number of these themes are analyzed in articles given to theoretical and conceptual formulations which offer new insights on our subject matter. In all of these, there is the recognition that migration and change do not, in themselves, constitute a problem. In the words of one of the authors, we cannot and should not try to prevent all forms of human mobility. In situations of change, most people survive and adapt. But for many, the experience of migration, transplantation, and relocation leads to uprooting and possibly to a lasting condition of uprootedness.

When migrants resettle into a new environment, they are usually exposed to a different culture, different ways of living and perhaps, to various forms of discrimination and prejudice. Previous research on migrant populations has shown that homesickness often persists along with an obdurate clinging to the past, thereby prohibiting successful adaptation to the present. Among people who have been oppressed in their home country, a lingering fear of the persecution may continue long after their migration.

Human service systems can perform vital tasks to assist migrant families and children in overcoming the trauma of uprooting and in resettling into a new environment. The successful resettlement of any migrant population requires of its members the ability to create a life which can span two worlds — the one they have just entered and the one they have left behind. Many are able to make the transition without external aid, but many others require help of the sort that is examined in papers in this volume concerning, among other things: the social policies and institutional practices of host societies regarding newcomers and foreign residents; the schooling and language training for children of immigrant families; and the provision of personal case services such as counselling and clinical treatment for the migrant who is psychologically distressed. These papers make it abundantly clear that the resettlement of migrant families and children involve variables at the societal and institutional levels as well as at the level of the individual and the family. In any large exodus of people, social, economic, and political factors are inherently involved and these, in turn, have important implications both for the community or society that receives migrants as well as for the community or society that loses the migrating population.

This volume was conceived following the 1977 Vancouver Congress of the World Federation for Mental Health, a conference which included workshop meetings on the themes of migration and innovative service programs for cultural minorities. With the site of the 1977 Congress on the west coast of Canada, it was appropriate to the setting that the workshops heard a number of reports on experiences involving people from the "Pacific Rim" and Southeast-Asian countries. In recent years, significant movements of population have occurred in that part of the world, with the most calamitous undoubtedly involving the tragic dislocation of refugees following the Vietnam conflict. Somewhat less dramatic has been a relatively large migration of people across the Pacific Ocean to North America, resulting not only from resettlement programs on behalf of Southeast-Asian refugees, but also from a marked increase in general immigration in this part of the world. Although there has been considerable study of European migration to the "New World", relatively little research has been given to the experiences of Asian immigrants in the United States and Canada. The latter is a focal point in several of the papers in this volume.

Two years after the Vancouver meetings, the World Federation for Mental Health convened again, this time in Salzburg, Austria, where a follow-up workshop on migration took place. Additional papers were contributed for this occasion and, because 1979 had been designated as The International Year of the Child, several of these works focussed on the particular problems experienced by the children of migrant families.

The papers contained in this volume are from the 1977 and 1979 Congress workshops. This is not the first occasion in which the World Federation for Mental Health has become associated with a publication on the subject of migration. In 1958, the topic of 'Uprooting and Resettlement' was the general theme at the Federation's eleventh annual meeting held in Vienna. The proceedings from the Vienna Congress were later published under the same theme-title.* Having the occasion now, over twenty years later, to follow up on the earlier work with this present volume of papers is indeed a rare opportunity.

The participants at the 1977 Congress workshops in Vancouver included Dr. Maria Pfister-Ammende, who had been one of the major contributors to the 1958 meetings in Vienna.** With her years of experience in working with refugees and immigrant groups under auspices of the United Nations and other organizations, Dr. Pfister-Ammende was given the task of opening the workshop meetings in 1977. Her comments are presented as a Prologue to the main papers in this volume.

There is, understandably, a mental health orientation in all of the papers. Their contents, however, reflect the perspectives of authors who come under a number of different professions and disciplines, including psychiatry, psychology, social work, education, and sociology. This is fitting inasmuch as the field of mental health is interdisciplinary, and professional interest in the phenomenon of uprooting and resettlement transcends the scope of any single field of activity or inquiry.

The contents in this volume are based on empirical observations of real-life events which should be of direct interest to persons working in all fields of human service that include immigrants or refugees among their clientele. Students in the various branches of social and behavioral sciences should also find the contents of this volume of interest because the data contained herein have relevance to their theoretical formulations on subjects such as human responses to changing environments and structures. Those with an interest in the general fields of multiculturalism and ethnic relations should also find these contents to be of immediate relevance.

In presenting this volume, I wish to express my acknowledgement and appreciation to all of the authors for their contributions. Special thanks are due to Roberta Beiser, Ann McCarthy, Susan Johnston and Nora Curiston in the Secretariat Office of the World Federation for Mental Health for their assistance in preparing the manuscripts; and to Dr. Tsung-yi Lin, the immediate

---

* World Federation For Mental Health, *Uprooting and Resettlement*, London and New York, 1960.
** Pfister-Ammende, Maria, 'Uprooting and Resettlement as a Sociological Problem', in *Uprooting and Resettlement*, WFMH, London and New York, 1960.

past-president of this organization, for providing the opportunity for me to come together with others who share a compassionate concern about the fate of the millions of migrant families and children throughout the world who are seeking a new life and a new home.

University of British Columbia RICHARD C. NANN
May, 1981

MARIA PFISTER-AMMENDE, M.D.*

PROLOGUE

Thank you for the honour of letting me present some introductory comments for this discussion on migration. My brief comments are based on experience in working with refugees and uprooted people, and on research into the problems of uprooting in different cultures.

Types of Migration and Mobility

Migration amd mobility can take various forms. They include:
  (1) Biological mobility occurs at different points in the life cycle, such as at adolescence, marriage, and retirement.
  (2) Sociological mobility occurs, for example, with the transfer of company executives from one country to another, or with the movement of staff employed in international organizations.
  (3) Voluntary and planned mobility may be motivated by a positive interest or may be economically induced. It is often associated with a country's use of foreign workers and, in other instances, with problems related to the "brain drain".
  (4) Forced planned mobility occurs when population groups must be removed, or a total community relocated, such as the relocation of about 250,000 people in order to construct the Aswan Dam in Egypt.
  (5) Forced unplanned mobility occurs usually as a result of political upheaval, for example, the situation with Vietnamese refugees. This type of movement involves high risks for the mental health of those people. In many cases, their reaction to this type of move will include a lingering fear of the persecutor which may be projected onto the new country, and be followed by depression, overt aggression, and apathy. Much later there may come an identity crisis of the next generation; the question "Who am I?"

Measures for Prevention of Uprooting

We must distinguish between primary and secondary prevention. To prevent migration itself is unrealistic but we must do what we can to alleviate the stress and strain leading to uprooting.

As far as *primary prevention* is concerned, the following principles are suggested:

*President, Schweizerisches Nationalkomitee für Geistige Gesundheit, and co-editor of: *Uprooting and After*, Maria Pfister-Ammende and Charles Zwingmann (eds.), New York, Springer-Verlag, 1973.

(1) Countries should produce the right skills in the right proportion to prevent a "brain drain" of their educated and skilled people.

(2) Migrant population groups should be actively involved in the planning of services to meet their needs; we should not be planning for such groups but planning together with them.

(3) Counselling services, as all other services, should be reachable.

(4) High risk groups include the single, the widowed, the old, the young male, and mothers without husbands. They should be sought out and special help provided to them since they are in particularly stressful situations.

(5) The participation of the receiving population is of paramount importance.

Secondary prevention of uprooting refers to provision of *early* assistance to already uprooted people. Here again the principles outlined under primary prevention would apply. We should bear in mind that we cannot and do not want to prevent all migration. We also cannot prevent all uprooting. But we should help to shorten its sufferings and assist uprooted people in finding new roots.

RICHARD C. NANN, D.S.W.

UPROOTING AND SURVIVING — AN OVERVIEW

People move for many different reasons. Human migration has been provoked by such diverse factors as war, natural calamities, industrialization and urbanization, persecution and discrimination, economic insecurity, professional ambition, and in the case of some individuals, just plain restlessness. In the Prologue, Pfister-Ammende presents a conceptual framework for classifying various types of migration and mobility. This is a very useful contribution because the typology serves, among other things, to differentiate mobility and change which are a normal part of human development or which serve a positive human interest, from other types of mobility which create a high risk for the health and well-being of the people involved.

The papers in this monograph touch on several types of human migration, involving populations in various regions of the world. Notwithstanding these differences, the common denominator which runs through this volume is change and its consequences for individuals, families, and communities involved in the transition. Perhaps the process of migration and resettlement was best described by Erik Erikson (1960), who had so aptly observed that migration is change; it is the transplantation of old roots and a search to find new roots in change itself.

This process is evident in the papers which follow concerning the resettlement of Vietnamese refugees in the United States (Lin *et al.*, Masuda *et al.*, Lourie). It is also of central interest in the several articles reporting on the experiences of immigrant populations respectively in North America (Ashworth, Nann, Yamamoto); in European countries (Verdonk, Stockfelt-Hoatson); and in Hong Kong (Mak and Chen). The process of transition and adaptation is of no less a concern to the author who examines the status of Turkish foreign workers in West Germany (Babaoglu); nor to the two writers who analyze the concept of culture shock and the phenomenon of "double-uprooting," as experienced by youths returning home after a stay in a foreign country (Coelho, Hoshino). And change, together with patterns of adapting to change, is certainly the main theme in the work examining the impact of industrialization and modernization on a rural West African population (Beiser).

The remaining papers in this volume are concerned with service delivery issues in the provision of help and assistance to migrant families and individuals (Li and Luk, Yamamoto, Lin, Chud, Nann and To). Here, also, change emerges as one of the central considerations. It is important that personnel in human service systems understand the transitional experiences of those whom they intend to help. Indeed, it is crucial that help-givers take into account the particular needs of a migrant population if assistance is to be of any use.

Notwithstanding the enormous stresses and strains which many migrants undergo, especially in cases where a move is involuntary, sudden and unplanned, one cannot help but be impressed by the resilience of human beings in coping with major change. Given the opportunity to resettle, most migrants will adapt and survive. However, adaptation may take many forms; some adaptive patterns can be described as healthy and successful, others less so. A major task for research, therefore, is to develop a better understanding of factors and conditions which bring about successful resettlement.

The papers in this volume contribute many important insights into the experiences of uprooting and resettlement. No attempt will be made to catalogue in this brief overview all of the important findings. However, some general observations are presented here.

RESETTLEMENT AS A SOCIAL ISSUE

The successful resettlement of immigrants and refugees is a complex process involving variables at the societal, institutional, family, and individual levels. The reasons which provoke a move, the personality makeup of the migrant, and the skills, knowledge and value systems he or she brings to a new environment are significant factors influencing the resettlement process. Equally crucial are the social, economic, and political policies of a receiving society which can serve either to facilitate or to frustrate the resettlement of newcomers. The contents in this volume include ample empirical evidence to show that hostile or inhospitable social policies and institutional practices lead to such deleterious consequences as unemployment or underemployment, poor housing, educational deficits in immigrant children, deviant behaviour, and mental health problems.

The needs of migrant families and children, therefore, cannot be dealt with in isolation from larger social, economic, and political issues. This point is obvious whether we are looking at Vietnamese refugees in the United States, Chinese immigrants in Canada or in Hong Kong, immigrant children in the Netherlands, families in rural West Africa, or families of foreign workers in West Germany.

A recurring theme which runs throughout this volume is the need for resettlement policies and practices which serve to keep families together. There is hardly a study of migrant groups that does not uncover great anxiety and concern over family members who have become separated, and an urgency to reunite with separated members.

As one specific example, anxiety over family separation and frustrations over the inability to do something constructive to help relatives still in the home country are cited as major contributing factors to problems of resettlement among Vietnamese refugees in the United States.

Allowing sufficient time for a successful transition to take place is another important need which is generally recognized but seldom incorporated into the social policies of receiving communities. The same research on Vietnamese refugees in North America shows that many persons in this group continued to exhibit instability in their lives which lasted into the third year of their resettlement and beyond. Under the best of circumstances, the successful transplantation of migrants to a new society seems to take at least three to five years.

LANGUAGE AND CULTURAL ROOTS

Acquiring proficiency in a different language is one of the first requirements of newcomers as they adapt to a new environment. Migrants must learn the language of their host culture or remain socially and economically disadvantaged. But this task is not merely one of memorizing a new vocabulary inasmuch as language cannot be separated from cultural values and norms. Learning a new language, therefore, means learning to be a part of a new social system, and this in turn may mean having to relinquish elements of the old.

Culture influences the adaptive strategies used by migrants as they begin life in a new environment. Their coping patterns have been learned within a previous cultural context and, as Coelho's account of Indian students in the United States would indicate, adaptive strategies which are suitable in a home environment may not be appropriate in a new environment. A similar observation is made by Yamamoto in his discussion of the Japanese in California. On the other hand, what is viewed as inappropriate or as a "problem" by members of a receiving society may often be due to a lack of cultural understanding. Coelho, for example, observes that many immigrants come from background environments where sadness, homesickness, and feelings of depression are not considered to be symptoms of a mental health problem.

Belief systems, values, and cultural roots run very deep. This should not be surprising when we consider that the cultural roots of people have evolved over centuries. In North America, as well as in other regions of the world with high rates of immigration, experience has shown that no matter how the dominant host society sets out to assimilate immigrants, cultural differences will persist. As an aside, this phenomenon seems to be acknowledged nowadays in Canada and in the United States, and whether one speaks of "multiculturalism" or of "cultural pluralism", the underlying policies constitute a sharp shift from a "melting pot" approach which, in North America at least, has been more of a myth than actuality. Whether addressed explicitly or implicitly, the importance of culture as a variable in adaptation and resettlement permeates all of the papers in this volume.

ETHNIC COMMUNITY AS SUPPORT SYSTEM

Among the social variables related to resettlement outcome, the nature and quality of social support seem particularly significant. One important source of such support is the presence of a relevant ethnic community (Murphy, 1977; Nann, 1977). In many immigrant receiving societies, the formation of ethnic networks has occurred with varying degrees of formalized structures. These may range from occasional gatherings on the part of some groups to highly developed ethnic institutional systems which can meet, more or less, all of its members' daily needs. In recent years, we have also witnessed the emergence of formally organized ethnic health and social service agencies (Lourie, Yamamoto, Nann and To).

As subsystems of a larger society, ethnic communities perform a number of important functions for their members, including maintenance of a cultural tradition, companionship, and protection against hostility and rejection. In addition to such general functions, the paper by Nann and To describes how an ethnic community support system can provide some very practical services for the new immigrant or refugee in areas such as; help in locating housing and employment, language interpretation and translation, connecting migrants with families still in the home country, and advice-giving and counselling.

Previous research (Murphy, 1977) has consistently found that where immigrants constitute a large proportion of the population, their relative rates of mental illness are lower than where they constitute a small percentage. The reason for this is still unclear. One explanation would be that the resources of the ethnic community provide a sufficient cushioning effect to the shock of resettlement into a new physical and cultural environment so that fewer symptoms of ill health will emerge than with groups who do not have similar access to an ethnic support system. There is, however, evidence to suggest a somewhat different explanation. The paper by Lin, for example, suggests that actual rates of disorder and illness may be more or less equal between a group imbedded in a strong ethnic support system and another group which lacks such a system. In the former case, however, problems of a very personal nature may be less likely to come to the attention of the larger culture's help-giving agencies, such as a mental health system, because of the ethnic community's ability to retain its members and to deal with their problems within the ethnic community itself. Despite the fact that our understanding of this matter is incomplete, the point remains that a relevant ethnic community is an important source of social support.

PERSONAL AND SOCIO-ECONOMIC VARIABLES

While resettlement may be a common task facing all members of a migrant group, different adaptive patterns will begin to emerge among members within the same group, and indeed, among members within the same family. The socio-economic background, the resources available, and the predispositions which individuals bring, will affect the adaptive outcome. Babaoglu's paper suggests that previous life experiences such as earlier moves either within or outside one's home country, can modify the resettlement experience. Factors such as age, sex, marital status, and educational and vocational background are also important variables. For example, the point is made in several papers

(Ashworth, Beiser, and Stockfelt-Hoatson) that the importance of literacy as an adaptive tool cannot be overemphasized.

Among a migrant population, female heads of households who are widowed, separated, or divorced experience the greatest amount of difficulties in resettlement. These mothers without husbands are often isolated not only from the main society but also from other members of their own migrant group.

Younger males, concerned with gaining their independence and manhood, can become greatly distressed over the difficulty of finding employment. Older males, conditioned to a well established role in the home country, may experience a great loss of social status when faced with the difficult task of learning a new language and the need to accept menial types of jobs. Their sense of humiliation is further aggravated when, as is often the case in a migrant population, wives must also take employment in order to make ends meet. Mental health workers are familiar with immigrant male patients who exhibit the syndrom of "status discrepancy".

The adaptive demands upon an adult female immigrant can be equally difficult. Apart from having to learn a new "woman's role" as defined by the cultural values of a host society, a significant number of mothers may find themselves isolated and shut in at home. This is particularly likely with mothers of very young children in a nuclear household. Moreover, human service workers in North America, for example, have become familiar with incidents of wife-beating among some immigrant families where the husband takes out his frustrations on a convenient target at home.

The children in a migrant population encounter their own special set of difficulties in the resettlement process. More often than not, it is the younger members of migrant families who have the greatest exposure to a new language and a new way of life through their formal and informal experiences in an educational system. While children are generally more quick to adapt to change, they are also the ones who are more likely to encounter an identity crisis later in life.

Whether voluntary or involuntary, and whether positively or negatively induced, the experience of uprooting and resettlement can be fraught with difficulties and upset. Symptoms of anxiety, depression, and homesickness are well-documented in various studies of migrant populations. Less is known about feelings of anger, irritability, and frustration. Overt anger and aggressive behaviour on the part of refugees or immigrants may be misinterpreted as a sign of ingratitude by members of a receiving society. However, constructive opportunities to express and to vent anger may be a necessary dynamic for successful resettlement to take place.

ECONOMIC ADAPTATION

One of the major tasks of refugees and immigrants is adaptation to the economic and financial setting of a receiving society. This is particularly challenging in cases of migrants from a rural economy background who resettle in a highly industrialized environment. Success in economic adaptation is dependent not only on the opportunities available to the migrant but also on his or her ability to manage the resources which are available for meeting immediate and long-range goals.

The migrant must make decisions about employment and financial security, and about the provision of basic necessities such as housing, food, clothing, and furnishings. The degree of current and future adaptation will be affected by the migrant's decisions in formulating goals and expectations, and by his or her ability to compete for employment. This in turn is influenced by factors such as; the existence and availability of jobs that can utilize the migrant's past training and work experience, opportunities for job-upgrading or re-training, language ability, and access to information about the labour market. If a relevant ethnic community system is present, a migrant may be able to meet immediate needs and expectations by securing employment associated with an ethnic industry. However, this may be at the cost of long range integration with the larger society's economic system.

Research findings reported in the papers concerning Vietnamese refugees in the United States indicate that underemployment is a major problem with this group. Most of the refugees are employed; yet a significant proportion still require public financial aid to supplement their low earnings.

EDUCATIONAL ADAPTATION

Education for children ranks very high among the resettlement goals of immigrant and refugee families, so that the school becomes for them a very important resource. Because of language and cultural differences, however, children of some migrant families find it extremely difficult to take advantage of educational opportunities.

As noted earlier, language learning and cultural adaptation are processes which are inextricably interwoven. The school experiences of immigrant children reported in several of the papers which follow indicate that adaptation to an educational system by immigrant children often brings on conflicts in the home between the younger and older generations. If adaptation and resettlement policies and programs are to consider the migrant family as the basic unit of concern, the experiences of immigrant children in school must be linked with family experiences in the home and vice-versa. In the final analysis, successful educational adaptation means that immigrant children must learn how to live comfortably between two cultures, the old and the new.

PLANNING AND DELIVERY OF RESETTLEMENT SERVICES

In many immigrant receiving countries such as Cannada, migrant populations are not adequately served by the traditional network of community educational, health, recreational, and social agencies (Head, 1977). In part, the reason is due to a highly bureaucratized and specialized structure of human service institutions. A number of important suggestions are presented in this volume's papers for improving the delivery of provisions and services to immigrants and refugees.

There is, first, the clear need to locate services where they are immediately and easily accessible to members of a migrant group. This often means the necessity of decentralizing programs to a local neighbourhood level. The multi-faceted nature of problems experienced by members of a migrant group will usually require the help of an interdisciplinary team, or of a well-coordinated set of programs. An essential ingredient is the use of bi-lingual personnel who can communicate in the language of the migrant group, and who understand its cultural background.

For example, when mental health services are required, the cultural background of the migrant group must be taken into account because it shapes attitudes toward mental illness and its treatment. Among some groups, the patient may be viewed as cursed, and the doctor as omnipotent. Placebo effects may be modified by culture, and treatment considered ineffective or insufficient if procedures such as injections have not been used (Nann and Seebaran, 1978). Different ethnic groups also show varying patterns in seeking help with mental health problems. Some may use a general medical practitioner for a long time, resisting psychiatric help until a problem becomes very serious. We see this very pattern among the immigrant Chinese both in North America and in Hong Kong as reported in the papers by Lin and by Mak and Chen.

Unlike their adult male counterparts who usually have a greater opportunity for contacts with the larger society because of pressures to earn a living, many immigrant women find themselves isolated and alone in the home. In families with young children in the home, a school-based program would be in a particularly good position to provide outreach services. Indeed, a school system would seem to be in a unique position to assist migrant families with children as, among the various societal human service institutions, it is the school which is most likely to have the broadest and most immediate contact. Moreover, if problems are encountered by members of an immigrant family, early manifestations will likely appear among children in school so that measures may be taken before the problems deteriorate. With the high priority given to their children's education, and a concomitant high regard given to a school system, migrant families are often more ready to accept services provided through this institution than those offered by some other governmental or non-governmental agency.

To emphasize a point made earlier in this overview, the cultural background of migrant families and children have important implications for those who are responsible for planning human service programs. In the field of mental health, for example, psychiatric therapy is alien to many immigrants and refugees. Some alternative approaches in the delivery of mental health services are examined in several of the papers which follow. One approach is characterized, generally, by a decentralized outreach service delivered by a professional multi-disciplinary team (Li and Luk, Lourie, Nann, Yamamoto). Another approach is described in the paper by Nann and To, which gives an account of a social-psychological support system indigenously organized and directed by members of an immigrant group themselves.

SOME RESEARCH ISSUES

Before concluding this overview, reference should be made to several research issues raised by writers who have contributed to this volume. The issues are mainly methodological but there is also an important substantive question. The latter concerns the matter of conceptual formulations underlying much of the reasearch on migrant groups which have tended to focus on what might be called the problems and pathologies of resettlement and adaptation. While none would argue against the need for better information about the difficulties experienced by migrant groups, there are at least two potential drawbacks if research is exclusively problem-focussed: The first is the danger that social change itself comes to be assumed as automatically "bad" for one's health and well-being; The second is the danger that significant variables and factors related to successful adaptation and resettlement may be ignored or missed.

Because the migrant groups of concern to us here can usually be culturally defined, it is important that research studies utilize measurements that are culturally relevant. This is particularly crucial in the field of mental health (itself a difficult concept to define) where the meaning and interpretability of many studies may be questioned on the grounds of the measures used. The study reported in the paper by Beiser is noteworthy because of the careful procedures taken to assure the cultural relevance of research instruments.

Lack of antecedent data about a migrant group is often another source of difficulty in the conduct of research on migration and resettlement. Use of retrospective data may at times be the only recourse but here, again, the meaning of findings must be interpreted with care. In this regard, one of the substantive issues of central concern to this volume is the question of whether mental health or illness is a determinant or an outcome factor in migration and resettlement. In a recent review of the relevant research literature, Klineberg (1979) came to the following conclusion: "no final answer was supplied to the difficult question of whether the amount of mental illness among immigrants is due to the trials they face, or to certain personal characteristics which occur more frequently among immigrants than among those who stay home." This issue is not resolved by the research findings contained in this volume, although there is the suggestion that important differences may exist between refugee and immigrant populations. For example, the studies of Vietnamese refugees in the United States concluded that many of their problems can be attributed to their refugee status. On the other hand, the reports on Chinese immigrants in Hong Kong and on Turkish workers in West Germany note the presence of significant numbers of persons who had experienced some form of psychological disorder prior to moving.

The length of time required for successful resettlement means that research in this area must be designed so as to measure change over a period of time. A longitudinal design is often used but this usually encounters the difficult task of maintaining contact with study subjects. It is well known that immigrants and refugees show a considerable amount of movement within a new country after they arrive. As a case in point, the researchers involved in the studies of Vietnamese refugees in the United States could locate only one-third of their original sample after a one-year period.

In spite of these and other methodological problems, ongoing research is required in order to improve and to expand our current knowledge about the process of migration and resettlement. This task will continue to be timely and urgent because we have come to realize that the uprooting of people is not a phenomenon which is of a temporal or transient nature. As Margaret Mead (1960) observed: "right through human history, we have had to solve difficulties initiated in one place by giving sanctuary in another."

Experience has shown that members of migrant groups have great capacity to adapt and survive. Adaptation patterns and resettlement outcomes, however, may be positive or negative when measured by the health and well-being of those who are in transition. In our current state of knowledge, the factors which modify the adaptive and resettlement experiences of migrant families and individuals are not completely known or well understood. It is hoped that the contents of this volume will serve both to increase our understanding, and to improve our ability to take effective action on behalf of those who have come among us in search of a new life and a new home.

REFERENCES

Erikson, Erik H.
    1960 Identity and uprootedness in our time. In: Uprooting and Resettlement, London and New York, World Federation for Mental Health.

Head, Wilson A.
    1977 Service accessibility and the multiracial community. In: Canadian Welfare, vol. 53, March-April.

Klineberg, Otto
    1979 An interdisciplinary and international perspective. In: Rokkan, Stein, (ed.), A Quarter Century of International Social Science, New Delhi, Concept Publishing Co.

Mead, Margaret
    1960 The place of mental health in the planning of immigration programmes. In: Uprooting and Resettlement, London and New York. World Federation for Mental Health.

Murphy, H. B. M.
    1973 Migration and the major mental disorders. In: Charles Zwingmann and Maria Pfister-Ammende (eds.), Uprooting and After, New York, Springer-Verlag.

Nann, Richard C.
    1977 Ethnic cultures and communities in North America. In: People and Places, Social Work Education and Human Settlements, New York. International Ass'n. of Schools of Social Work.

Nann, Richard C., and Seebaran, R.
　1978 Migration: uprooting and surviving. In: Beiser, M. *et al.* (eds.), Today's Priorities in Mental Health: Knowing and Doing, Miami, Symposia Specialists.
Nann, Richard C. and Ben Chud
　1981 Mental health of children of migrants and cultural minorities. In: Stuart H. Fine *et al.* (eds.), Today's Priorities in Mental Health: Children and Families – Needs, Rights, and Action, Dordrecht, Holland, Reidel Publishing Company.

KEH-MING LIN, M.D. MINORU MASUDA, Ph.D., and
LAURIE TAZUMA, M.D.

PROBLEMS OF VIETNAMESE REFUGEES IN THE UNITED STATES

INTRODUCTION

The extrme difficulties in adapting to a new socio-cultural environment have long been recognized and repeatedly discussed. Psychiatric problems have been observed to be more prevalent among immigrants than in a native-born population (Odegaard, 1932), and refugees or displaced persons seem to be in particularly high risk as evidenced by numerous case reports and several clinical studies of various refugee groups since the end of World War II (Pedersen, 1949; Edwards, 1956; Eitinger, 1959; Mezey, 1960; Meszeros, 1961; Eitinger and Grunfeld, 1966; Tyhurst, 1971; Chu, 1972; Rumbaut and Rumbaut, 1976). Paranoid reaction, depression, anxiety, reactive psychosis, and coversion reaction have been observed as particularly prevalent. A marked tendency of somatic over-concern and increased incidence of somatic complaints were also found to be present in several refugee groups (Eitinger, 1959; Tyhurst, 1971). Increase in incidence of physical health problems has been reported in Chinese expatriates and Hungarian refugees (Dohrenwend *et al.*, 1974). However, most of these studies were based on retrospective clinical material. Questions about the extent of influence of the adaptational difficulties on health and mental health status of the refugees, factors which contribute to adaptation and health, and the characteristics of high risk subgroups among the refugees, have hardly been explored. In this era of community mental health, these seem to be highly relevant issues to be investigated.

The significance of refugee problems can readily be appreciated by the fact that, according to a United Nations report, an estimated 45 million persons have been denied residency in their homeland from 1945 to 1967, and in 1968, alone, 7 million people were considered international refugees (United Nations, 1969). According to this same report, there are today about 15 million refugees in the world.

People with refugee experiences are scattered in every corner in today's America, forming segments of population groups requiring special health and mental health consideration. The collapse of the South Vietnam regime in April, 1975 brought another surge of refugees into the United States. In subsequent months, more than 140,000 Vietnamese fled their homeland and entered the U.S.A. They started to arrive in the Greater Seattle area as early as May, 1975. In early June, two local community agencies, namely the Employment Opportunity Center (EOC) and the Asian Counselling and Referral Service (ACRS) proposed a multifaceted program called 'Project Pioneer' (EOC, 1975; ACRS, 1975). This program was promptly funded by federal, state and private sources and started offering courses and counselling with the purpose of easing the transition of the Vietnamese into American life.

Perceiving the need for health service and research, the University of Washington Department of Psychiatry and Behavioral Sciences formed a team on a volunteer basis. A health clinic was set up within the context of 'Project Pioneer' and operated for six months, from July through December, 1975. The project was designed from its inception to be a longitudinal yearly follow-up, using observation and questionnaire administration to document the health and mental health statuses of the refugees in different stages of adaptation. Phase I of this study was conducted in combination with health services (Lin, 1976). Phase II of this study, completed one year later, was conducted by home visits. During the total period of this research, the authors have had extensive contact with the Vietnamese communities as well as with many helping agencies in the Greater Seattle area, frequently serving as consultants for the psychosocial problems of the refugees.

METHODS

Phase I of the study, conducted in the context of 'Project Pioneer', recruited clients non-selectively from sponsoring agencies in the community as well as from state-sponsored agencies. Questionnaires were administered to the clients during the course of basic hygienic and everyday medical knowledge classes, with the help of Vietnamese interpreters.

Phase II was conducted through home visits by the same research team consisting of a male Chinese psychiatrist, a female Japanese American medical student, and an experienced Vietnamese community worker. Interviews, observation, and administration of questionnaires were done in an atmosphere of concern for the health and welfare of the refugees, usually with maximal cooperation elicited.

Among the 152 subjects of Phase I, 54 were seen again in Phase II. The remainder of Phase II subjects came from two sources: 39 subjects who did not participate in the Phase I study were randomly sampled from 'Project Pioneer' and 48 were newly recruited from the Vietnamese community. Total subjects for Phase II numbered 141 (Table I).

Due to the voluntary nature of participation and the high mobility of the refugees in the first year of resettlement, the samples were not entirely selected at random; furthermore, not all Phase I subjects were included in the Phase II follow-up. However, the characteristics of the subjects were very similar to each other for both phases (Table I).

The instruments used included the Cornell Medical Index (CMI), the Social Readjustment Rating Questionnaire (SRRQ), the Schedule of Recent Experience (SRE), and a questionnaire for health and social history especially designed for this study. They were all translated into Vietnamese by a group of Vietnamese overseas students and double-checked by a competent Vietnamese doctor.

TABLE I
Characteristics of Study Subjects

		Phase I (N = 152)	Phase II (N = 141)
Sex	Male	66%	68%
	Female	34%	32%
Age	Below 21	23%	17%
	21–30	40%	53%
	31–45	23%	22%
	46–65	14%	9%
	Over 65	1%	1%
Marital Status	Married	42%	44%
	Widowed	2%	6%
	Divorced/Separated	4%	2%
	Never Married	52%	48%
Education Level	Grade School	14%	4%
	High School	53%	49%
	Technical School	0	1%
	College	30%	43%
	Graduate School	3%	2%
Religion	Buddhist	57%	50%
	Catholic	19%	27%
	Protestant	13%	14%
	No Preference	11%	9%

The data derived from the SSRQ and the SRE will not be described here, but are presented in a companion article which immediately follows this paper (Minoru Masuda *et al.*, 'Life Changes among Vietnamese Refugees'). The CMI is a widely used health questionnaire consisting of 18 sections totalling 195 questions. The first 12 sections (A–L) deal with symptoms in discrete physiological systems while the last 6 sections (M–R) are mainly concerned with psychological symptomatology. Since the appearance of the CMI in 1949, many studies conducted in various cultures have found this instrument to be a valid screening tool for neurotic tendencies and a sensitive indicator of a person's physical and mental health (Brodman *et al.*, 1956; Brown and Fry, 1962; Chu and Rin, 1970).

The health and social history questionnaire was designed to obtain information about current health needs, personal and family medical history, family constellation, habits, attitudes and perceptions about the refugee experience, employment status, training and employment history, social activities, contacts with Vietnamese, contacts with Americans, agency utilization and English proficiency.

Based on the questions on family constellations and supplemented by personal interview findings, four family types were identified, comprising the following: Type I – young single men who have no relatives in this country; Type II –

individuals who live with nuclear family units; Type III — individuals who have extended family networks in this country; and Type IV — women, divorced or separated, who are also heads-of-households (Table II).

TABLE II
Types of Families

Type	Description	Phase I	Phase II
I	Single young male alone	9 (17%)	24 (18%)
II	Small family units	30 (55%)	75 (57%)
III	Large family units with extended network	12 (22%)	28 (21%)
IV	Divorced or widowed female head of household	3 (6%)	5 (4%)

Three social contact indices were constructed from the health and social history questionnaires: (A) Vietnamese community contact index; (B) American society contact index; and (C) helping agency contact index (Table III).

TABLE III
Social Activity Indices

A. Vietnamese community contact index (Scale of 0–17):

small social gatherings	0–3
large social gatherings	0–3
number of Vietnamese good friends	0–3
Vietnamese neighbors	0–3
reading Vietnamese publications	0–1
listening to Vietnamese radio	0–1
belonging to Vietnamese associations	0–1
knowledge of Indochinese Service Center	0–1
contact with Vietnamese community worker	0–1

B. American society contact index (Scale of 0–21):

small social gatherings: Caucasian	0–3
small social gatherings: Asian	0–3
large social gatherings: Caucasian	0–3
small social gatherings: Asian	0–3
good friends, non-Vietnamese: Caucasian	0–3
good friends, non-Vietnamese: Asian	0–3
relation with sponsor	0–2
adaptation to American food	0–1

TABLE III (continued).

C. Agency contact index (Scale of 0–7):

Indochinese Service Center	0–1
Employment opportunity Center	0–1
International District Health Center	0–1
Asian Counselling & Referral Service	0–1
Asian Community Health Center	0–1
Vietnamese community worker	0–1
Voluntary agency service	0–1

RESULTS

As can be seen in the data presented in Table I, the refugee population is fairly young. About half of the study subjects were still unmarried; most had at least high school education and were previously employed in Vietnam. Religious preferences were predominantly Buddhism; Catholicism came next, and then Protestantism, representing recent Western influence. The mean CMI scores for Phase I are presented in Table IV; as are the CMI scores, according to sex/age categories, marital status, and family types. The only difference between males and females that reached statistical significance is found in the M–R scores.

TABLE IV

CMI Scores and Their Relationships with Various Sample Characteristics. Phase I (N = 152)

Age	A–L Male	A–L Female	M–R[a] Male	M–R[a] Female	A–R Male	A–R Female
21	25	18	14	20	39	39
21–30	22	23	10	16	32	38
31–45	20	20	9	12	29	32
46–65	21	21	10	5	31	26
All ages	22	22	10	15	32	37

Marital Status	A–L	M–R	A–R
Married	21	11	32
Never married	22	13	35

Family Types	A–L	M–R	A–R
I	15	11	26
II	25	16	41
III	19	10	29
IV	24	22	46

	A–L	M–R	A–R
TOTAL CMI SCORES	22	12	34

[a] $F = 2.24$, $p < 0.01$; this is the only comparison that reached significance.

The CMI total scores of Phase II are very similar to those of Phase I. However, the influence of different variables on the CMI scores in Phase II is significantly different. As can be seen in Table V, the interaction between age and sex is significant in all three CMI categories.

TABLE V
CMI Scores and Their Relationships with Age and Sex. Phase II (N = 141)

	A–L		M–R		A–R	
TOTAL CMI SCORES	22		13		34	
Male/Female	M	F	M	F	M	F
21[a]	24	14	13	9	37	23
21–30[a]	18	30	10	19	28	49
31–45[a]	18	27	10	20	28	48
46–65[a]	33	22	16	14	49	36
All ages[b]	22	26	13	17	34	42

[a] Age-sex interaction: A–L: $F = 3.98, p < 0.01$
  M–R: $F = 4.97, p < 0.005$
  A–R: $F = 4.94, p < 0.005$
[b] Male/female differences: A–L: $F = 4.69, < 0.05$
  M–R: $F = 12.31, < 0.001$
  A–R: $F = 8.15, p < 0.005$

There is also a trend for married people to have higher scores than singles, a trend which reaches significance when a chi-square test is used (Table VI and VII).

TABLE VI
Distribution of High A–R Scores (> 30)
in Relation to Marital Status

	A–R (> 30)	A–R (< 30)
Married	35	27
Never Married	27	40

$\chi^2 = 3.37, p. = < .05$

TABLE VII
Distribution of High M–R Scores (> 10)
in Relation to Marital Status

	M–R (> 10)	M–R (< 10)
Married	39	23
Never Married	29	38

$\chi^2 = 4.97, p. = < .05$

Phase II CMI scores also differ significantly among the four family types (Table VIII): the widowed/separated female heads-of-households (Type IV) have the highest scores; and the single, young male (Type I), the lowest.

TABLE VIII
Relationship between CMI Scores and Family Types. Phase II

Family Type	N	A–L	M–R	A–R
I	24	17	9	26
II	75	22	13	36
III	28	24	12	37
IV	5	36	23	60
F		2.64	2.96	3.10
P		=0.052	<0.05	<0.05

In Phase II, the possible effects of employment status and various social conditions on CMI responses are also examined. These include emplyment status, English proficiency, mode and means of transportation, and status of public assistance. Among these variables, the presence of public assistance is the only factor significantly related with higher A–R as well as M–R scores (Table IX).

TABLE IX
Relationship between CMI Scores and Various Employment and Social Conditions in Phase II

	n	A–L	M–R	A–R
Currently employed	71	21	12	32
No	55	24	13	38
Driver's license	88	21	12	32
No	37	25	14	39
Own car	61	20	11	32
No	66	24	14	38
English proficiency				
Good	12	18	8	26
Poor	115	23	13	36
Public Assistance	76	24	14[a]	38[a]
No	48	18	10[a]	28[a]

[a] $p < .05$

None of the three contact indices correlates significantly with any of the CMI scores.

The CMI profiles for the two phases (Figure 1) are quite similar to each other. In the somatic category (A–L), Phase II has somewhat lower scores in Sections D (GI symptoms), F (skin symptoms) and H (GU symptoms); and higher scores in sections E (musculoskeletal symtoms), I (neurological symptoms), J (illness behaviors), and L (habits). In the psychological category (M–R), Phase II has higher scores in sections N (depression), Q (hostility and irritability); and lower scores in M (anxiety).

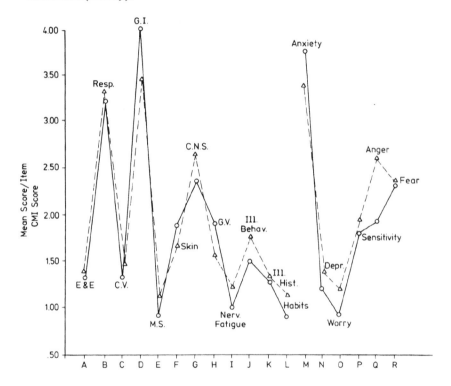

Fig. 1. Mean category score profile – CMI. Phase I ○———○ (1975); Phase II △------△ (1976).

DISCUSSION

Difficulties in adapting to a new socio-cultural environment, especially for those with no preparation for such a major change, are tremendous and multifaceted. The dramatic life changes refugees are forced to make undoubtedly will have an impact on the psychological as well as physical health statuses. During our more than two years' contact with the Vietnamese refugees, we have witnessed feelings of homesickness, grief over the losses incurred during the process of evacuation or fleeing, uncertainty about the future, and endless incidents of frustration. Clinically, we have seen many Vietnamese suffering from various forms of psychosomatic symptoms accompanying general feelings of nervousness and sadness which persisted into the second year of their arrival. This impression is, to a certain degree, confirmed by the CMI findings of both phases of this study: the CMI scores of both phases are much higher than the norms in the US and UK. Brown and Fry (1962) suggested 30 for the total (A—R) scores, and 10 for the psychological (M—R) scores as cut-off points for probable emotional difficulties. Using these criteria, 52% and 56% respectively of the Vietnamese refugees fall into this category. This clearly demonstrates the extent and degree of distress these people experienced in the first two years of their life in the host culture.

It could be argued that this apparent elevation of CMI scores might reflect the socio-cultural differences between Americans and Veitnamese rather than the effect of refugee status. This is a reservation which must be considered while interpreting the data, since there is no CMI data available on Vietnamese prior to their coming to the U.S.A. However, in a study of Chinese in Taiwan, a population with an Asian background, similar economic development, and a similar political situation, the CMI norms were much closer to the above-mentioned Western norms (Chu and Rin, 1970). Using the Chinese norms for comparison, the CMI socres in the Vietnamese refugees would still be alarmingly high. It appears most probable that cultural factors played only a minor part, and the refugee status was mainly responsible for the elevation of the CMI scores in this case. This should be no surprise since the detrimental effects of changes in socio-cultural environments, including migration, temporary displacement, immigration, and refugee condition on both mental and physical health have been demonstrated time and again in the past. Chu and Rin (1970) found that among displaced persons recently come from mainland China to Taiwan, the CMI scores were significantly higher than among native Taiwanese (also Chinese in origin).

The fact that total CMI scores stayed essentially the same for both phases merits further discussion. Mathers (1974) suggested a "gestation period" of approximately two years for identity change to happen after entering a new environment. Hong and Holmes (1973) reported that a three year period is necessary for reasonably successful adaptation to occur in an individual who held professional status before migration. Holmes and Masuda (1973) indicated that illnesses frequently clustered around the two year point after the occurrence of major life changes. The CMI data in the second phase of this study provide further supportive data for this previously observed slowness of the adaptation process.

The high correlation of the CMI findings in the two phases suggests that people vary in their styles of adaptation to a new environment, and that those responding with high symptomatology initially tend to maintain a high symptomatology later. A report by Rahe *et al.*, (1978) on a mental health survey in Camp Pendleton reveals elevation of CMI scores very similar to our data. Evidently, the ordeal of the Vietnamese did not start immediately after they settled in this area. The tasks to be learned and the stresses encountered may differ at various stages of adaptation, but the nature and severity of stress are quite similar and will continue until their readjustment to the new environment reaches a reasonably comfortable stage. In some cases, this adaptation may be accomplished within a few years, yet in others it may take a lifetime.

Breaking down the sample into subgroups according to demographic characteristics and family types reveals interesting results. An almost universal character of the CMI data is that scores for females are higher than scores for males, with the ratio around 3.2 in all three categories.

In Phase I, there is no correlation between the CMI scores and any other variables such as age, marital status, family type, education and occupation. Contrary to this, in Phase II, significant differences are found in age, sex, marital status, and family type. The implication of this change from Phase I to Phase II seems to be that the initial tasks dealing with adaptation and stress are basic and affect refugees indiscriminately. One year later, after the refugees had become more settled in their new environment, factors associated with less favorable adaptation start to emerge. The effects of family types, age groups by sex, and marital status found in Phase II will be discussed below.

Among the four different family types, the divorced/widowed female heads-of-households (Type IV) appear to be the least resourceful and most distressed. They are usually quite isolated, not only from the main society, but also from other Vietnamese. The same condition had been noticed among Cuban refugees (Rumbaut and Rumbaut, 1976). The extreme elevation of the CMI scores clearly confirmed the interview impression that they were overwhelmed by the situation and acutely in need of help. This is not a minor problem since, according to the HEW Report (1976), about 1,300 (10% of the refugees) belong to such a family type. Contrary to our original speculation that the 15% Vietnamese without any relatives in the US (usually male ex-servicemen, Type I), would fare worse because of lack of social support, many of these seem to be able to hold jobs, establish new relationships with other Vietnamese, and Americans to some extent, and have CMI scores which are the lowest of the four family types. Types II and III, people with small and large family units, responded to the CMI similarly, with scores intermediate to Type I and IV. It is possible that the Type I subjects benefited from having less responsibility and more free energy to adapt to this highly individualistic, often fast changing society.

With respect to age and sex, CMI scores are higher in older (over 46) and younger (less than 21) males and reproductive-age females (21–45). The case for the older men is not difficult to understand, for most of them had been well established in Vietnam, while in this country they became the most disadvantaged when learning a new language, acquiring new skills and getting meaningful jobs relative to their status and expectations. This is not so with older females, since their roles as housewives, mothers of grown-up children and grandmothers are not fundamentally different from their roles in Vietnam. This observation confirms the concept that "status inconsistency" is a major detrimental factor to the health status of immigrants, as suggested by Abramson (1966). One possible explanation for the fact that women in their reproductive years have higher CMI scores, and by inference, are most distressed, is that they not only have to learn how to be housewives, mothers, and women in this new environment, but quite frequently, they must also try to find jobs or go through training programs because of the urgent financial needs of the family. Thus, they must adapt to several new roles simultaneously.

One speculation that may account for the fact that males in their late teens tend to be more distressed than females of the same age would involve role expectations. For example, the males are concerned about making a living while female, often still living at home, are protected from the direct impact of stress. Another possibility might be that the stereotypes of American society are more favorable to young Asian females, often viewed as feminine and adorable, than to young Asian males, frequently seen as weak and non-masculine (Bolen, 1977).

In a recent study of 14 Chinese-speaking Vietnamese heads-of-households (Yamamoto *et al.*), Zung depression scale scores were found to correlate to employment status. This kind of correlation is not present in Phase II of our study when CMI scores are compared to employed status. This discrepancy might be due to the different scales used: Zung's scale covers only intrapsychic depressive feelings and the vegetative depressive signs, while the CMI covers all aspects of psychological and physical symptomatologies. The former (i.e., the Zung scale) may better reflect the current status of a person's affect, while the latter (or CMI) reflects more accurately the long-term feeling of well-being. Furthermore, several factors may have undercut the beneficial effects of employment: firstly, it is our impression that most of the jobs held by the refugees were temporary and highly unstable; secondly, it is clear that among those employed, the majority held menial jobs which might boost the mood initially, but in the long run would prove to be a humiliating condition of "status inconsistency".

In sharp contrast to this, the acceptance of public assistance is directly related to the CMI scores, with those receiving public assistance showing more symptoms. This indicates that people on public assistance may be less resourceful and less healthy.

It has been suggested that social isolation is a most taxing problem for the immigrants/refugees. Ruesch *et al.* (1948) suggested that every effort should be made to help those with greater potential to integrate into the host society, while for those with less potential, efforts should be directed at increasing their contacts with people from the same culture, thereby forming a supportive subculture for better social interaction and mutual support.

For the purposes of our study, we formulated three indices of refugee social contacts: contact with Vietnamese; with Americans; and with helping agencies. None of these indices correlated to the CMI scores, (although they correlated to each other). The reason for the lack of correlation between CMI scores and indices of social contact is not clear; it could be that many factors, such as age, sex, employment status, etc., tend to contaminate these two indices. Hence, they did not represent the socialization or acculturation factors effectively. The profile scores of the CMI sections for both phases reveal some interesting points. Some of the differences in the somatic sections could be partly due to the abrupt change of physical environment, such as increased incidence of traveller's diarrhea in Phase I, etc. The differences in the psychological part suggest that, when the Vietnamese first arrived, anxiety symptoms prevailed. One year later, having become more or less comfortable with the immediate environment, the refugees became less anxious, but feelings of frustration and homesickness were accumulating. Based on this finding, one might anticipate an increasing incidence of depressive problems among the refugees; problems which, paradoxically, tend to become more severe when the refugees seem better conditioned to their surroundings. Tyhurst (1971), studying refugees from Eastern Europe, came up with a similar observation, i.e. that it took several months for the refugees to experience "psychological arrival", and then they became susceptible to the full impact of the situation. Since success in adapting to a new environment invariably involves losing old attachments and gaining new identities, in some ways the experience might be comparable to going through a grief reaction. We might speculate that the process of adaptation could be divided into stages of denial, anger, depression and finally, acceptance. Further research in this area would be of great help in our understanding the nature of depression and other psychiatric problems in these people.

The most notable CMI difference lies in section Q which deal with feelings of anger and irritability. In the one year lapse between Phase I and Phase II, scores in this section went up 34%. This increase may be due both to the lessening of inhibition and to the accumulating feelings of frustration. It has been suggested by Meszaros (1961) that hostile, aggressive attitudes in refugees are not necessarily destructive. Having observed 100 refugee clients, Meszaros discerned five basic adaptive styles: the two most successful styles involved either severe criticism and anger at the host society or at fellow refugees. Despite these critical attitudes, these refugees continued to absorb and assimilate new information and make progress; they fared better than those who were overinhibited, emotionally paralyzed, or despairing. If this is the case, then the recognition, understanding and encouragement of expression of angry feelings which are bound to be pervasive and intense, would be of great help to the refugees in facilitating their adaptation processes.

REFERENCES

Abramson, J. H.
 1966 Emotional disorder, status inconsistency and migration. American Journal of Public Health, February, 23–48.

Bolen, J. S.
 1977 The Asian woman psychiatrist. Paper prepared for the Task Force of Asian-American Psychiatrists, March.

Brodman, K., Erdmann, A. J. Jr., and Wolff, H. G.
 1956 Manual of Cornell Medical Index-Health Questionnaire, New York Hospital and the Department of Medicine (Neurology) and Psychiatry, Cornell University Medical College, revised.

Brown, A. C. and Fry, J.
 1962 The Cornell Medical Index-Health Questionnaire in the identification of neurotic patients in general practice. Journal of Psychosomatic Research 6: 185.

Chu, H. D.
 1972 Migration and mental disorder in Taiwan. In: W. Lebra (ed.), Transcultural Research in Mental Health, Honolulu, East-West Center Press.

Chu, H. M. and Rin, H.
 1970 The distribution of psychiatric symptoms in a Chinese community: An application of modified Cornell Medical Index-Health Questionnaire in a psychiatric epidemiological study. Journal Formosa Medical Association 69: 29–44.

Dohrenwend, B. S., Dohrenwend, B. P. (eds.)
 1974 Stressful Life Events: Their Nature and Effects, New York, John Wiley and Sons.

Edwards, A. T.
 1956 Paranoid reactions. Med. J. Aust. 1: 778–779.

Eitinger, L.
 1959 The incidence of mental disease among refugees in Norway. Journal of Mental Sciences 105: 326–338.

Eitinger, L., Grunfeld, B.
 1966 Psychosis among refugees in Norway. Acta Psychiat Scand 42: 315–328.

Employment Opportunities Center (Seattle)
 1975 Project Pioneer: Employment Opportunities Center, Seattle, Wa., June. (mimeographed)

HEW Refugee Task Force
 1976 HEW task force for Indochina refugees. Report to the Congress, June.

Holmes, T. H., and Masuda, M.
 1973 Life change and illness susceptibility. In: Separation and Depression, J. P. Scott and E. C. Senay (eds.), Washington, D.C., American Association for Advancement of Science, No. 94.

Hong, K. E. M. and Holmes, T. H.
 1973 Transient diabetes mellitus associated with culture change. Archives General Psychiatry 29(11): 683–687.

Lin, K. M.
 1976 Vietnamese Health Clinic: Summary Report. Department of Psychiatry and Behavioral Sciences, University of Washington, Seattle, Wa., March. (mimeographed)

Mathers, J.
 1974 The gestation period of identity change. British Journal of Psychiatry 125: 472–474.

Meszaros, A. F.
 1961 Types of displacement reactions among the postrevolution Hungarian immigrants, Canadian Psychiatric Association Journal 6: 9–19.

Mezey, A. G.
   1960 Psychiatric illness in Hungarian refugees, Journal of Mental Science 106: 628–637.
Mezey, A. G.
   1960 Personal background, immigration and mental disorder in Hungarian refugees, Journal Mental Science 106: 618–627.
Odegaard, O.
   1932 Emigration and insanity: A study of mental disease among the Norwegian-born population of Minnesota. Acta Psychiatr. et Neurol. Supplement IV.
Pederson, S.
   1949 Psychopathological reactions to extreme social displacements (refugee neuroses). Psychoanalytic Review 36: 344–354.
Rahe, R. H., Looney, J. G., Ward, H. W., Tung, T. M., Liu, W. T.
   1978 Psychiatric consultation in a Vietnamese refugee camp. American Journal of Psychiatry 135: 185–190.
Ruesch, J., Jacobson, A. and Loeb, M. B.
   1948 Acculturation and illness. Psychological Monographs: General and Applied 62(5): 1–40.
Rumbaut, R. D. and Rumbaut, R. G.
   1976 The family in exile: Cuban expatriated in the United States. American Journal of Psychiatry 133(4): 395–399.
The Asian Counselling and Referral Service (Seattle)
   1975 Social Service Program to Complement Project Pioneer. Asian Counselling and Referral Service, Seattle, Wa., June. (mimeographed)
Tyhurst, L.
   1971 Displacement and migration: A study in social psychiatry. American Journal of Psychiatry 107: 561–568.
United Nations
   1969 Refugee Report.
Yamamoto, J., Lam, J., Fung, D., Tan, F., and Iga, M.
   Chinese-speaking Vietnamese refugees in Los Angeles. Preliminary Draft, Department of Psychiatry, University of Southern California, Los Angeles, California.

MINORU MASUDA, Ph.D., KEH-MING LIN, M.D., and
LAURIE TAZUMA, M.D.

LIFE CHANGES AMONG THE VIETNAMESE REFUGEES

INTRODUCTION

In the previous paper, we described our longitudinal studies on Vietnamese refugees, and examined their health and mental health statuses based on the administration of the Cornell Medical Index.* The results indicate that the refugees are at great risk of illness as they attempt to cope with a strange culture.

In this paper, we present data concerning life stresses experienced by the same group of refugees at two administrations of test instruments — on their arrival to the United States in 1975 (Phase I), and a year later in 1976—77 (Phase II). Since we have already described the characteristics of the study population, we will not repeat those here except to say that, in general, the subjects were young, with more than half below the age of 30 at the time of our studies; two-thirds were male; one-half were unmarried; and they were generally a well-educated group as half had finished high school, and more than one-third had gone to college.

METHODOLOGY

The three questionnaires administered to the refugees which will be discussed in this paper are: The Social Readjustment Rating Questionnaire (Holmes and Rahe, 1967); The Schedule of Recent Experience (Hawkins *et al.*, 1957; Rahe *et al.*, 1964; Holmes and Masuda, 1973); and the Cornell Medical Index (Brodman *et al.*, 1956).

The Social Readjustment Rating Questionnaire (SRRQ) was developed by Holmes and Rahe as a means of quantifying the perceived amount of psychosocial readjustment required to cope with a series of life events. Some 43 life events were distilled from the clinical experiences of over 5,000 patients as having an association with the onset of illness. The method, derived from psychophysics, has been established as a valid psychometric instrument (Stevens, 1975).

From the self-report SRRQ, a scale is derived — the Social Readjustment Rating Scale (SRRS). The scale scores used here are based on the geometric mean (Masuda and Holmes, 1967).

There are many cross-national studies utilizing the SRRQ for elucidating similarities and differences in cultural perceptions of life events. These studies

---

* K. Lin, M. Masuda, and L. Tazuma, 'Problems of Vietnamese Refugees in the United States'.

have compared the American SRRS to scales derived with subjects from other countries such as Japan (Masuda and Holmes, 1967); Western Europe (Harmon *et al.*, 1970); Spain (Celdran, 1970); San Salvador (Seppa, 1972); Malaysia (Woon *et al.*, 1971); Cuba (Valdes, 1976); Denmark (Rahe, 1969); Sweden (Rahe *et al.*, 1971); and New Zealand (Isherwood, 1976). The high correlation in rank ordering of life events as found in these studies is also highlighted by differences in magnitude estimations which have been explained on cultural bases.

The Schedule of Recent Experience (Hawkins *et al.*, 1957; Rahe *et al.*, 1964; Holmes and Masuda, 1973) is a self-report retrospective recall record of the occurrence of the SRRS life event items on a periodic basis, e.g., here for the calendar year. Developed in conjunction with the SRRQ, use of The Schedule of Recent Experience (SRE) and the SRRS allows for a calculation of annual life change units according to the formula:

$$\text{Life Change Units (LCU's)} = \Sigma \text{ (Item Occurrence} \times \text{Item Score)}.$$

There is considerable evidence (Holmes and Masuda, 1973) that links the accumulation of life change to the onset of illness — the greater the magnitude of life change, the greater the risk of illness, and furthermore, the greater the seriousness of the chronic illness (Wyler, Masuda and Holmes, 1971).

The concept of life events impacting on individuals to produce a variety of illnesses has been extended to their association with other behaviours such as academic performance of students (Valdes and Baxter, 1976); and teachers (Carranza, 1972); as well as job performance (Clinard, 1973). Life change has been associated with traffic accidents (Selzer and Vinokur, 1974); incarceration of criminals (Masuda *et al.*, 1974); children's psychobiological adjustments (Coddington 1972; Padilla *et al.*, 1976); and injuries to football players (Bramwell *et al.*, 1975).

The Cornell Medical Index (Brodman *et al.*, 1956) is a 195-item self report symptom questionnaire. The symptoms are distributed among 18 categories, A through L, featuring psysiological systems; and M through R, featuring psychological symptomatology.*

RESULTS

The Social Readjustment Rating Scale (SRRS)

It is of interest to compare the 1976 Vietnamese SRRS to the American SRRS (Figure 1). The American data are based upon a previously studied sample of

---

* A description of the Cornell Medical Index categories is given in the previous paper, Lin *et al.*, 'Problems of Vietnamese Refugees in the United States'.

394 middle-class subjects (Masuda and Holmes, 1967). The rank order correlation between the two SRRS's is highly significant 0.72 (p = < .001), indicating that the Vietnamese refugees generally perceive life event items in a fashion similar to the Americans.

However, as Figure 1 indicates, there are considerable differences in the mean score of individual items. In general, items which are in the upper third of American scoring tend to be scored lower by the Vietnamese. Items such as "death of a spouse"; "divorce"; "major personal injury or illness"; "being fired from work"; "marital reconciliation"; "retirement"; "gain of a new family member"; and "change in health of a family member"; were given high scores by the Americans. In the middle third scoring range, the scores are similar except for two items which the Vietnamese scored significantly higher. These are: "foreclosure of mortgage"; and "outstanding personal achievement". In the lower scoring range, the Vietnamese tend to exhibit higher scores than do the Americans. These included items such as: "change in church activities"; "mortgage loan less than $10,000"; "change in family get-togethers"; "change in eating habits"; and a tremendously different score for "minor violations of the law".

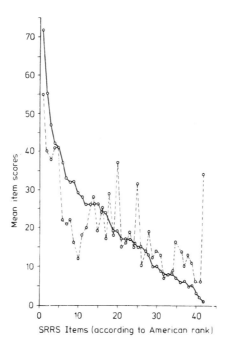

Fig. 1. SRRS: American and Vietnamese (1976). ○────○ American; ○─ ─ ─○ Vietnamese. r_s = .716 (p < .001).

The SRRS's for the Vietnamese in 1975 and in 1976 are compared in Figure 2. Here, each SRRS was graphed according to its own item ranking. It is immediately apparent that one year after their arrival, the perceptions of the refugees have become uniformly reduced. The rank order correlation of items between these two phases (r_s), is 0.90; a higher correlation coefficient, as might be expected, than between American and Vietnamese SRRS.

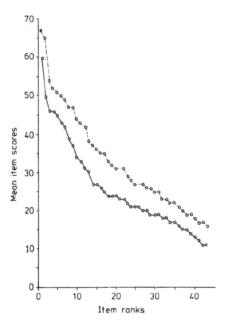

Fig. 2. Vietnamese SRRS (1975 and 1976). ○——○ 1976; ○— — —○ 1975. r_s = .902 (p < .001).

Life Changes

Annual life change units in the refugee population over a five year period are shown in Figure 3. The pre-evacuation Vietnam years (1972–74) show consistently low mean annual life changes. The traumatic events of the 1975 evacuation and movements are reflected in a roughly fourfold increase in life change as compared to pre-evacuation. The 1976 column represents an incomplete year compilation (average of nine months), but is shown here, nevertheless, to indicate that almost a year after their arrival, life changes continued to remain high.

It is relevant to try to probe the sources of problems of the Vietnamese inasmuch as continued high life change indicates a continued need for psychosocial readjustment. In looking at the individual life event items in terms of their frequencies of occurrence, we find decided differences between the years 1975 and 1976. In order to facilitate exposition of these differences, the 43 life events were categorized according to items related to work, spouse, family, etc. (Masuda and Holmes, 1978). When the mean frequencies of the items in each of the categories are summed and divided by the number of items in the category, it is apparent that the category mean frequencies did not change in a similar fashion; some fell in 1976 to almost pre-evacuation levels (e.g., personal); some fell significantly from the peak in 1975, but continued to remain high (e.g., life style); while others continued and surpassed the peak of 1975 (e.g. work).

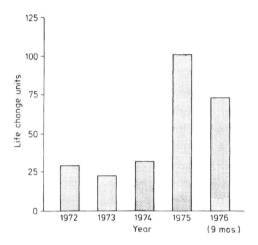

Fig. 3. Life Change Units: Vietnamese refugees.

The three divergent groups of category frequencies are shown in Figure 4. Financial and life style problems continue to plague the refugees; and events related to work, spouse, troubles with the law, and schooling have continued even higher than in the turmoil year of 1975.

The correlation of life change units to the total CMI (Health Status) scores (A–R) for Phase I and Phase II are shown in Table I. There is a weak but positive and significant correlation between life changes and health status. There is a stronger correlation exhibited in Phase I when evacuation and acute resettlement were in progress.

DISCUSSION

Cross-cultural studies with the Social Readjustment Rating Scale (Holmes and Masuda, 1973; Masuda and Holmes, 1978) have shown that there is a universality in the manner in which people rank order the significance of life events. It is also

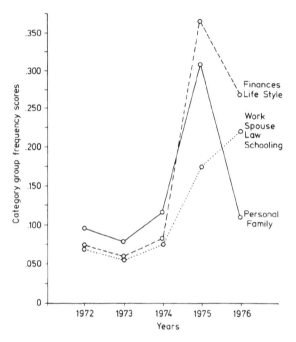

Fig. 4. Vietnamese SRE item frequency.

TABLE I
Correlation of Life Change Units and Total CMI Scores

	Correlation Coefficient (r)	P
Phase I (79)	0.27	< .01
Phase II (127)	0.15	< .05

true that there is variability in the strength of these rank order correlation coefficients, with higher correlations obtained among Western countries, while those societies which are of the Third World (e.g., Asian, Central and South America) have lower correlation coefficients when compared to the American SRRS. Thus, the perceptions of the Vietnamese refugees are in agreement with the previous observations.

The fact of reductions in magnitude estimation of life events one year after the first administration of the SRRQ is a new and unexpected finding. It suggests that, in the turmoil year of 1975, when evacuation, movement, survival, relocation and living problems were acute and immediate, the situation of flux had engendered a psychological state so as to heighten the perceptions of the meaning of life events. A similar kind of phenomenon had been noted by Janney *et al.* (1977) in their study of two Peruvian towns; one devastated by an earthquake, the other physically unharmed. A comparison of these two groups of town people in their SRRQ responses showed clearly, one year after the earthquake, that the catastrophe-affected people had higher scores. These data would indicate that the situational and psychological set of individuals can, and does, affect their perception of life events, especially as it might relate to a highly unusual and traumatic catastrophic series of events (such as forced overseas migration and earthquake devastation).

The accumulation of relatively high life changes by the Vietnamese during 1975, the year of evacuation, is to be expected. However, the continuingly high accumulation in 1976 reflects the difficult process of coping and adjusting to American society, and survival in it. The continued experiencing of life events tells of the multitude of perceived changes that are ongoing in the lives of the Vietnamese, and presages further difficulties in their adjustments. Rahe *et al.* (1978), using a modified SRE, found that life changes in the six-month period immediately prior to leaving Vietnam varied according to age and sex. Men between the ages of 20 and 39 recorded the greatest number of life changes, while the lowest were recorded by women 40 years of age and older.

However, these difficulties, as evidenced by life event occurrences, are not evenly distributed. Events of a personal nature (three items — e.g., "change in family get-togethers"; "trouble with in-laws"; "change in health of family member") fell from a high in 1975 to almost pre-1975 levels, indicating relative stability in these areas. The categories of life events related to finances and changes in life style, although falling below the 1975 level, remain high and were the highest of all categories. Life events related to finances comprise five items and include, for example, "change in financial state"; "business readjustment". Life events related to life style comprise nine items and include, for example, "changes in sleeping, eating and personal habits"; "change in social and church activities"; "change in residence"; etc. An even more interesting group of four categories of life event items are those which, in 1976, continue as high as in 1975 and/or even higher in occurrence. These four categories are related to work (six items, e.g., "troubles with boss"; "change in work conditions"; "change to different line of work"; etc.); to spouse (seven items, e.g., "arguments with spouse"; "marital separation"; "wife beginning or stopping work"; etc.); to law (two items, "jail detention" and "minor violations of the law"); and to schooling (two items, "change in schools" and "begin or end school").

Continuing changes in life events as seen in the Vietnamese distribution give an indication of the areas in which the refugees find instability, (i.e., in work, finances, spouse relations, life style). Social and mental health programs focussing on these areas would presumably ease the Southeast Asian refugee adjustment.

The positive correlation found between accumulated life changes and health status as evidenced by the Cornell Medical Index is supportive of the generalization that the greater the amount of life change experiences, the greater the risk of illness. The CMI is useful as a diagnostic aid and screening instrument and has predictive value in risk for mental health. In Part I (Lin et al., 1979), the high CMI scores demonstrated by the Vietnam refugees implied a serious jeopardy to their current health. The data presented in this paper indicate that the continued occurrence of life events is implicated in that high risk state.

REFERENCES

Bramwell, S. T., Masuda, M., Wagner, N. D., and Holmes, T. H.
- 1975 Psychosocial factors in athletic injuries: Development and application of the Social and Athletic Readjustment Rating Scale (SARRS). Journal of Human Stress 1(2): 6–20.

Brodman, K., Erdman, A. J., Jr., and Wolff, H. G.
- 1956 Manual of Cornell Medical Index-Health Questionnaire. New York Hospital and the Departments of Medicine (Neurology) and Psychiatry, Cornell University Medical School. Revised.

Carranza, E.
- 1972 A Study of the Impact of Life Changes On High School Teacher Performance in the Lansing School District as Measured by the Holmes and Rahe Schedule of Recent Experience. Ph.D. Dissertation, Michigan State University, College of Education, East Lansing.

Celdran, H. H.
- 1970 The Cross-Cultural Consistency of Two Social Consensus Scales: The Seriousness of Illness Rating Scale and the Social Readjustment Rating Scale in Spain. Medical Thesis, University of Washington, Seattle.

Clinard, J. W.
- 1973 Life change events as related to self-reported academic and job performance. Psychol. Rep. 33: 391–394.

Coddington, R. D.
- 1972 The significance of life events as etiologic factors in the diseases of children. II, A study of normal population. Journal of Psychosomatic Research 16: 205–213.

Harmon, D. K., Masuda, M., and Holmes, T. H.
- 1970 The Social Readjustment Rating Scale: A cross-cultural study of Western Europeans and Americans. Journal of Psychosomatic Research 14: 391–400.

Hawkins, N. G., Davies, R., and Holmes, T. H.
- 1957 Evidence of psychosocial factors in the development of pulmonary tuberculosis. American Rev. Tuberc. 75: 768–780.

Holmes, T. S. and Masuda, M.
- 1973 Life change and illness susceptibility. In: Scott, J. P. and Senay, E. C. (eds.), Separation and Depression: Clinical and Research Aspects. American Association for the Advancement of Science, Washington, D. C., Publication No. 94.

Isherwood, J. and Adams, K. S.
- 1976 The Social Readjustment Rating Scale: A comparative study of New Zealand and Americans. Journal of Psychosomatic Research 20: 211–214.

Janney, J. G., Masuda, M., and Holmes, T. H.
- 1977 Impact of a natural catastrophe on life events. Journal of Human Stress 3(2): 22–34.

Lin, K. M., Tazuma, L., and Masuda, M.
  1979 Adaptation problems of the Vietnamese refugees. Part I: Health and mental health status. Archives of General Psychiatry 36(9): 955–961.
Masuda, M. and Holmes, T. H.
  1967 The Social Readjustment Rating Scale: A cross-cultural study of Japanese and Americans. Journal of Psychosomatic Research 11: 227–237.
Masuda, M., Cutler, D. L., Hein, L., and Holmes, T. H.
  1974 Life events and prisoners. Archives of General Psychiatry 131: 903–906.
Masuda, M. and Holmes, T. H.
  1978 Life events: Perceptions and frequencies. Psychosomatic Medicine 40(3): 236–261.
Padilla, E. R., Rohsenow, D. J. and Bergman, A. B.
  1976 Predicting accident frequency in children. Pediatrics 58: 223–226.
Rahe, R. H., Meyer, M., Smith, M., Kjaer, G., and Holmes, T. H.
  1964 Social stress and illness onset. Journal of Psychosomatic Research 8: 35–44.
Rahe, R. H.
  1969 Multi-cultural correlations of life change scaling: America, Japan, Denmark, and Sweden. Journal of Psychosomatic Research 13, 191–195.
Rahe R. H. Lundeberg, U., Bennett, L., and Theorell, T.
  1971 The Social Readjustment Rating Scale: A comparative study of Swedes and Americans. Journal of Psychosomatic Research 15: 241–249.
Selzer, M. L. and Vinokur, A.
  1974 Life events, subjective stress, and traffic accidents. American Journal of Psychiatry 131: 903–906.
Seppa, M. T.
  1972 The Social Readjustment Rating Scale and the Seriousness of Illness Rating Scale: A comparison of Salvadorans, Spanish and Americans, Medical Thesis, University of Washington, Seattle.
Stevens, S. S.
  1975 Psychophysics: Introduction to its Perceptual, Neural, and Social Prospects. New York: John Wiley and Sons.
Valdes, T. M. and Baxter, J. C.
  1976 The Social Readjustment Rating Questionnaire: A study of Cuban exiles. Journal of Psychosomatic Research 20: 231–236.
Woon, T. Masuda, M., Wagner, N. N., and Holmes, T. H.
  1971 The Social Readjustment Rating Scale: A cross-cultural study of Malaysians and Americans. Journal of Cross-Cultural Psychology 2: 373–386.
Wyler, A. R., Masuda, M., and Holmes, T. H.
  1971 Magnitude of life events and seriousness of illness. Psychosomatic Medicine 33: 115–122.

NORMAN V. LOURIE, M.S.W., D.H.L.

INNOVATIVE MENTAL HEALTH SERVICES FOR INDO-CHINESE PEFUGEES IN THE UNITED STATES

INTRODUCTION

The research literature reveals that experiences involving the sudden uprooting and migration of populations have been accompanied by extreme and often lingering physical, psychosomatic and social stress. It may be expected, therefore, that the Indo-chinese who have settled in the United States face a broad range of both acute and chronic problems of identification and adjustment. Whether forced or voluntary, the precipitous departure from home and homeland has evoked anxiety and insecurity inherent in the new and unknown. The sense of isolation and abandonment felt by many Indo-chinese are exacerbated in the face of the unpredictable avalanche of social, vocational and economic problems. Apathy, depression, disappointment, anger and other psychological aspects of stress can be experienced along with a range of psychosomatic complaints. The Indo-chinese Immigration and Refugees Assistance Act of 1975 created the Department of Health, Education and Welfare's Task Force for Indo-chinese Refugees. For the Federal fiscal year ended September 30, 1980, the national government appropriated $516,900,000 to care for refugees who arrived. To bring refugees into the United States the cost was $207,295,275 in that year. In the comments which follow, a brief description is given of the current status of the refugees, and of a variety of new projects and programs which have been established to serve the refugees. In the U.S. the national government pays 100% of resettlement costs for up to three years. From 1975 to 1980, 415,225 Indo-chinese refugees were admitted to the U.S.

INCOME SUPPLEMENT

Over 45% of the refugees are receiving at least part of their support from federally funded refugee cash assistance in August 1980.

EMPLOYMENT

Labor force participation rates of the Indo-chinese refugees aged 16 years and older show an increase with length of time in the country according to the November 1980 survey.

Refugees; entered 1975	74.4% male and 51.6% female
USA Population in general	77.4% male and 51.6% female

UNDEREMPLOYMENT

While the resettlement program's primary efforts have been directed toward obtaining employment and self-sufficiency for refugee families, a large number of families remain unemployed. Although 74.4% of the males who arrived in 1975 are employed, 11.8% are receiving some type of federal cash assistance supplementation.

EDUCATION

In one year $18.5 million were provided to local school districts for the education of refugee children. Another $10.25 million were provided for project grants to state and local education agencies for adult refugee education. Other funds supplemented these expenditures.

STATUS

All legally admitted refugees can become permanent residents and then citizens. Legal aliens receive all citizen benefits.

FAMILY REUNIFICATION

A growing frustration among refugees, individually and collectively, is over their inability to do something constructive to help relatives who are separated. This frustration over family separation has been a growing contributing factor to problems of resettlement and adjustment, and is viewed by many as a further cause for depression and psychological strain among the refugees.

NATIONAL MENTAL HEALTH PROJECTS

Psychiatric therapy is alien to the Indo-chinese culture, and the Indo-chinese tend to stigmatize mental health problems. The language barrier has also inhibited effective treatment. A number of National Demonstration Projects were funded to explore potential approaches to the mental health problems of the Indo-chinese. Following are some examples:

Project A

A $20,000 grant to the Department of Mental Health, in the state of Massachusetts, funded a team composed of a social worker and a paraprofessional to make site visits to each of the six New England states in order to review the cases of refugees identified as having mental health problems by clergy, agencies and sponsors. The team has developed information which can be helpful in the design of other mental health programs for Indo-chinese refugees, and has lent permanence towards efforts to help mental health systems to realistically address the needs of refugees and to pass along the information to agencies, sponsors, and providers of social services.

Project B

The Refugees Mental Health Project, Columbus, Ohio, called together the resettlement offices of six states for a two-day workshop on mental health problems among the refugees. The workshop discussion centered on how best to provide proper mental health services to the refugees, especially those with severely urgent needs for assistance.

Project C

In Denver, Colorado, a six-member team consisting of a Vietnamese paraprofessional, a psychologist and five Asian Americans (one psychiatrist, two psychologists, a social worker and a public nurse) completed a six-months project, treating 50 Indo-chinese families and designing a comprehensive plan for delivery of mental health services to the refugee population in Colorado.

Project D

The International Institute of San Francisco, under a $68,000 grant, completed a year long project to provide training services in three counties to refugees who were trained as mental health paraprofessionals.

Project E

The Asian Counselling and Referral Service in Seattle, Washington, under a $20,000 grant, utilized a toll-free telephone line, public service radio and TV announcements as means of making the service known to refugees settling in that area. Audio tapes were also developed to help professional counsellors to reach refugees effectively.

STATE PROGRAMS CATEGORICALLY DESIGNED FOR INDO-CHINESE REFUGEES

Some states have established categorical services for Indo-chinese refugees. These include:

Wisconsin

The Resettlement Assistance Office is to: (1) develop and maintain comprehensive information on all available services; (2) link, through a referral procedure, the refugees, sponsors and volunteer agencies with the appropriate services; (3) follow up and determine whether the referral service was actually delivered; (4) through public education, promote an awareness of the information and referral service, and an understanding of the resettlement process, i.e. (a) coordinated public education, (b) toll-free number for information sharing, (c) printing and circulating bilingual newsletters.

California

Agencies working with Indo-chinese refugees in California are finding that an increasing number of mental health problems are surfacing. Depression, anxiety reactions, and psychosomatic disorders are common. Less common, but evident, are suicides; husband, wife and children abuses; and marital conflicts caused by separation. There have been manifestations of maladjusted children. Finally, a number of schizophrenia and paranoia cases have surfaced.

These mental health problems are believed to be arising from the following conditions: (1) separation of family members during the evacuation; (2) lack of preparation for the evacuation; (3) decisions that were, of necessity, hastily made at the time of evacuation; (4) the unlikelihood of being able to return safely, if at all, to their homeland; (5) underemployment, or no employment; (6) cultural differences; (7) inability to speak English, and scarcity of persons in the American society speaking the Indo-chinese languages; (8) lack of Indo-chinese "community"; (9) inadequate housing; (10) uncertainty about the future and their status. In order to serve the comprehensive mental health needs of the Indo-chinese, a pilot project was designated to: (1) identify the incidence of mental health problems among the Indo-chinese refugees; (2) develop a Demonstration-Pilot Program for training paraprofessionals to assist professionals dealing with mental health problems; (3) provide linkages between the refugees and mental health services; (4) assist mental health agencies in relating to the problems of the refugees and thereby helping to reduce the number of severe mental health cases; (5) disseminate to the refugees information about mental health services.

Louisiana

Through the Associated Catholic Charities in the city of New Orleans, the following refugee services are given:

1. *Employment Services*

   (a) Exploration and assessment of employment needs of individual clients.
   (b) Assessment and employment potential and aptitudes of clients.
   (c) Individual and group counselling in procedures for securing and maintaining employment.
   (d) Referral to, and arrangement with, prospective employers on behalf of the clients to develop specific job opportunities for that particular individual.
   (e) Interpreter on job-site when deemed necessary.

2. *Health Related Services*

(a) Exploration and assessment of health needs, medical service arrangements and mental health referrals.
(b) Medical education to familiarize refugees with home health care, and to ensure that the refugee understands and follows through on health programs.
(c) Maintaining central files on each client's progress and problems.
(d) Developing and using bilingual video-taped lessons for teaching health education to clients, and preparing bilingual health care handbook.
(e) Interpreter available on a 24-hour basis for emergencies.

3. *Home Management Services*

Training is given in all areas of household management via individual and family counselling sessions. Skill areas include:
(a) Management of household budgets.
(b) Use of common household equipment and proper cleaning techniques.
(c) Consumer education.
(d) Nutrition and food preparation, safe cooking and storage methods.

4. *Housing Improvement Services*

(a) Assisting in locating suitable housing.
(b) Making repairs to homes.
(c) Working with landlords to upgrade substandard housing.
(d) Assisting in purchasing or renting of homes.

5. *Education and Training Services*

Arranging for placement in high school, college, vocational training, or conversational classes.

6. *Family Counselling Services*

Intake, diagnosis, and initial determination of treatment is made upon referral. Whenever feasible, group work is used. Tapes listed below are sometimes used in group discussions.
(a) Different cultural attitudes toward aging.
(b) Coping with grief and loss, as in separation from family and homeland.
(c) Raising children in USA.
(d) Short job service announcements prepared for weekly 30-minute program in Vietnamese on Sunday mornings.

Pennsylvania

The Office of Mental Health trains staff on awareness of the cultural adjustment process experienced by the refugees so that:

(1) adjustment problems may be dealt with at an early stage before they become debilitating emotional problems;

(2) inappropriate referrals are avoided in the mental health system;

(3) mental health staff know where to turn within their area for information and consultation regarding Indo-chinese referral.

Training is also provided to Indo-chinese professionals and paraprofessionals.

CONCLUSION

The circumstances surrounding the immigration of the Indo-chinese to the USA have been unique in many respects. The varied and continued study, assessment and treatment of this new population of American society is continuing. Most significant is the emergence of ethnic professional societies and mutual assistance groups which specialize in dealing with mental health problems in their own populations. American mental health groups are becoming more sensitive to ethnic issues and continue to train their staffs in special cultural and ethnic mental health matters.

JOE YAMAMOTO, M.D.

BEGINNING AN ASIAN/PACIFIC MENTAL HEALTH CLINIC

INTRODUCTION

As misfortune may at times lead to some good, the downfall of the Resthaven Community Mental Health Center in Los Angeles led to a decision by the County to fund a small Asian/Pacific Mental Health Clinic. The Resthaven Community Mental Health Center was adjacent to Chinatown near the center of the city of Los Angeles. As a community mental health center, the Resthaven had been challenged by the Asian communities and most especially by the Chinese-Americans to provide relevant bilingual and bicultural services.

For a number of reasons, including the discontinuation of the Federal Staffing Grants for community mental health centers, the Resthaven Community Mental Health Center had to close its doors. A result of this was the freeing up of County funds supplied through the Short Doyle Act (90% by the State of California and 10% by Los Angeles County). Approximately $ 200,000 of the funds budgeted for the Resthaven Community Mental Health Center came to be earmarked for an Asian/Pacific Mental Health Clinic.

The Asian-American Mental Health Training Center and, more specifically, the Affiliated Asian-American Mental Health Task Force, had been advocating the initiation of an Asian/Pacific mental health clinic for at least a year prior to this situation. Thus, in parallel with the bankruptcy of the Resthaven, the efforts of the Asian-American Mental Health Task Force Led to this decision by the Los Angeles County Mental Health Department and specifically, the Central Health Services Region. With this decision, the change in funding from contracts with the Resthaven Community Mental Health Center to the initiation of a wholly County-funded and managed clinic was made. The process took same time and it was not until April 1, 1977 that personnel could be hired.

LANGUAGE NEEDS AND STAFFING

Prior to the official clearance to use the budget funds, the Asian-American Mental Health Task Force and I, as the Director Designate to the Asian Mental Health Clinic, had been meeting to plan the staffing pattern of the clinic and to review priorities for services. Based on our past experience in the field, it was recommended that eight Asian/Pacific languages be covered. In addition, the members of the Asian-American Mental Health Task Force were acquainted with mental health professionals, most specifically psychiatric social workers who could speak varbus Asian languages and thus, recommended a staffing pattern which included a number of psychiatric social workers. The language included

Chinese, Japanese, Korean, Filipino, Vietnamese, Samoan, Guamanian and Thai (or Laotian or Cambodian).

In order to try to be as inclusive as possible, the initial staff hired have included a Korean mental health psychologist, a Chinese physician, a Japanese-speaking nurse counsellor, a Filipino psychiatric social worker and a Samoan psychiatric social worker. The clerical staff included a Filipino typist clerk and a Korean stenographer. A vietnamese typist clerk was also hired who spoke Cantonese, Mandarin, and Vietnamese. Thus, with both professional and clerical staff, many of the Asian languages to be served were covered. Recruitment of an additional three professionals (one nurse counsellor, and two psychiatric social workers) was temporarily postponed. After a period of time, because of the number of Korean patients seen in our clinic, it was decided to add a Korean psychiatric social worker. The remaining openings are being reservedwhile we search for professionals who can cover Vienamese, Gumanian, and Thai (or Laotian or Cambodian).

PROBLEMS OF LOCATION

In preparing for a suitable site for the clinic, it was decided that an area close to downtown Los Angeles would be appropriate. We decided on purpose not to have it set in Chinatown, little Tokyo, or Manila Town. The reason for this was that we wanted to be identified more broadly as an Asian/Pacific Mental Health Clinic. As it turned out, it was also important that the Clinic be located in the district of the County Supervisor where the Resthaven Community Mentel Health Center had been functioning. So, for all of these reasons, the search for a suitable site centered in an area approximately a mile and one-half from the City Hall of Los Angeles.

For various reasons, an attempt was made to affiliate with the already established Asian groups. For example, the first site was on the same floor as the Asian Community Service Center. Here, there were County and CETA employees who spoke many of the Asian languages which we hoped to cover. Unfortunately, this site was leased by another agency and was lost to us. Subsequent searches have included a site adjacent to the Asian-American Mental Health Training Center, a long established and pioneering effort to train professionals to work in the mental health field. This is a federally granted unit which has increased the number of mental health workers of diverse Asian/Pacific backgrounds.

While the rather frustrating search for a suitable site was being carried out, there were several false starts, with sites being deemed unsuitable or unavailable or having already been leased. In the meantime, plans have continued to find an appropriate location.

EDUCATIONAL AND MEDIA CAMPAIGN

The Asian/Pacific Mental Health Clinic has been temporarily located in borrowed quarters at the Los Angeles County USC Medical Center in the Psychiatric Outpatient Clinic building. Although the space is limited, a decision was made to proceed with the educational campaign for the various ethnic communities. The reason for this decision was clear evidence in the County Department of Mental Health statistics showing that Asians underutilized mental health services. In Los Angeles County, the following is true: Blacks overutilize mental health services; Whites tend to use about their proportion; the Spanish-speaking population use a bit more than half their proportion of mental health services; and Asian/Pacific Islanders underuilize mental health services even more than the Spanish surnamed. Priority was, therefore, given to the education of the community and professionals who serve as gate-keepers to mental health services. For example, we wanted to contact health professionals, the Ministry, social workers and others who work with Asian/Pacific Islanders. In addition, a media campaign was planned. This included public service announcerment spots for television and radio, and brief announcements in the ethnic newspapers. This campaign is at present going on so that I am unable to report the final results, although gradually patients have been referred and seen by the Asian/Pacific Mental Health team.

As a result of this education campaign, we expect the initial cases to include a number of chronically ill and mostly severely psychotic patients who have been kept at home and taken care of by their families (Lam, 1976).

As a part of the education and information campaign in the various Asian/Pacific communities, and to overcome the disadvantage of the prejudices of Asians against mental health services, it was decided to emphasize non-psychotic issues. We felt this was important in making the path towards appropriate mental health services easier. Thus, the campaign will emphasize issues such as: (1) tension symptoms; (2) insomnia; (3) psychosomatic complaints, including hypertension; (4) specific interpersonal problems, such as marital problems and family discord; and (5) problems of self-development, including male/female role conflicts resulting from the culturally learned roles and expectations of Asians which conflict with those prevalent in the American culture. Psychiatric labeling of patients in a pejorative sense will be de-emphasized by this focus on the problems of tension symptoms, psychosomatic disorders and other non-psychotic issues. In order to provide the best possible services, considerable effort will be spent towards appropriate and culturally relevant diagnostic procedures.

OVERCOMING USER RELUCTANCE

In order to circumvent the great reluctance of Asian/Pacific Islanders to use psychiatric services, not only will the services have to be made more palatable through a de-emphasis of such issues as psychotic labeling, but services which are flexible and available in the local communities will also be necessary. Some background to this is quite relevant.

Among the most recent immigrants (the Koreans and Vietnamese), the State of California has funded two groups who have been working in the community. One group, focussing on Vietnamese refugees, has been funded through the International Institute of Los Angeles. Here, Vietnamese "Uncle" counsellors have been seeing their clients in their homes. This is a very time consuming and expensive way to proceed. However, they have found that the Vietnamese refugees will not seek services in the standard facilities. Numerous attempts have been made to refer patients, and relatively few have succeeded as referrals.

It is the rare person who has been personally brought by a counsellor or helper to our Outpatient Clinic at the LA County USC Medical Center, and who then has been seen by a psychiatrist. Although the referrals have been on the order of five times the number who actually do come to the Clinic, some of the people are being seen, and we hope, helped by the counsellors in their homes.

The second case involves a Korean group, where a grant was given to the Korean Mental Health Center presently located in a church in the community. This counselling group has had numerous meetings with the members of the community and offers a wide spectrum of counselling services. Again, they do not have a mental health clinic in the sense of guidelines using the medical model; rather, they have counsellors under the supervision of a person with a doctorate in Psychological Political Science. Nevertheless, in offering services in the community, an unmet need has been served. It is expected that some of these clients at the Korean Mental Health Center will also be referred and be seen in a formal clinic setting. However, there will remain some who will only come to a less structured and "unofficial" counselling center.

With this background then, the rationale is seen for the assignment of the Asian Mental Health Clinic team in various ethnic communities. Our hope is that the County of Los Angeles will approve a plan for the assignment of clinic members in the various ethnic communities on a part-time basis. One example is the stationing of a Chinese (Cantonese-speaking) professional person at the Chinatown Service Center, which is a multi-service facility. This service centre receives a small grant from the Lutheran Church to offer counselling services. These services are given to teenagers, for example, who need counselling. Our mental health professional may serve as a back-up mental health consultant. In addition, should there be patients seen at the Chinatown Service Center who seem to require more definitive mental health evaluation, it is our hope that the County will permit this to be done on the site with due registration of the patient.

Similar examples are also important with regard to the Korean community. We hope that one of our Korean-speaking mental health professionals will be able to spend part of his time at the Korean Mental Health Clinic at the aforestated church. Other examples are outreach in the Japanese community both at Little Tokyo Towers and at the Japanese Retirement Home; in the Samoan County facility in the city of Carson; and in the Filipino Community Center in central Los Angeles. When required by clinical conditions, home visits will be made.

PSYCHIATRIC STATUS SCHEDULE

Because of the many languages and cultures that we confront with our patients, we decided to use the Psychiatric Status Schedule (PSS) of Spitzer, Endicott and Cohen (1968). Briefly, this is a highly structured psychiatric examination schedule which, in the English Version, is provided as a ring-bound booklet and a convenient answer sheet. There are some 321 items which the clinician is asked to score as being either true or false. Many of the items have to do with answers to questions such as: poor appetite, sleep disturbance, and concern about physical health. In addition, there are items which are related to the examination of mental status. Examples are: insight, remote memory, orientation, grooming, quality of speech, emotion and attitude toward interviewer. The reason for the decision to use the PSS was the convenience and the previous computerization of the material. The PSS is convenient in that the answer form can be used for the examination regardless of the culture and language of the patient. That is to say, we now have translations into Japanese, Chinese, and Korean. In addition, translations into Vietnamese, Samoan and Tagalog are progressing. The clinician can score the PSS answer sheet in whatever language the patient speaks. The answer sheets can then be placed upon the English language booklet and others who do not speak the language of the patient can see what the responses are.

In addition, we have initiated an audio-visual version of the PSS in different languages, including slides in English, Japanese, Korean and Chinese. I also have a brief audio tape with the same questions in the four different languages.

Eventually, we hope that every patient seem in the Asian/Pacific Mental Health Clinic will have the PSS done in the appropriate language. In addition, where it is possible, we hope to have the MMPI which has already been translated into Chinese, Japanese and Korean. We do, of course, expect to use appropriate normative criteria such as those suggested by James Butcher in his book *A Handbook of Cross-National MMPI Research* (Butcher, 1976). This, then, would be a positive step forward towards more appropriate diagnoses of Asian/Pacific Islanders.

TREATMENT FOR ASIAN/PACIFIC ISLANDERS

Consideration of culturally relevant treatment for Asian/Pacific Islanders must include an understanding and empathy about the family relationships in the diverse groups. As an example, I would like to use the case of the Japanese culture and Japanese-Americans. But first, I must preface my remarks with a caveat. We must constantly assess the generation, ethnicity, social class, geographical area of residence, and historical era during which the Asian/American patient under consideration has migrated to the United States and has experienced American acculturation processes. Many of these issues have been discussed by Gordon (1946) and also by Kitano (1969).

With this awareness of the differences among Japanese-Americans in terms of their generation, social class, area of residence, and time of immigration to the United States, we can then initiate a discussion of the least acculturated group. Our premise is that those who are most acculturated would tend more generally to fit the traditional Western psychotherapeutic methods. Those who are unacculturated will need therapeutic methods which are tailored to their backgrounds and needs.

As Nakane has pointed out in her book *Japanese Society* (1970), the Japanese grow up in a highly structured and hierarchical society. Everyone is either superior or inferior to oneself. This begins with the family where the roles of the father, mother and each child are clearly defined. For example, the roles of the children are defined in ter ms of sex and age. In the Japanese language, there are no words to denote a sister or brother, only words which designate older brother or younger brother or older sister or younger sister. This is specifically understandable in the context of the vertical society. In addition, Japanese are socialized to place great important on social interactions in relationships and less emphasis on individuality. This has been well described by Takie Sugiyama Lebra in her book, *Japanese Patterns of Behaviour* (Lebra, 1976).

Lebra points out that the Japanese develop a sense of identity through group belongingness. Thus, for all their lives they belong to their parental family, the school family, the work family, or professional family, and this is an enduring sense of identity. Indeed, in the Japanese culture there is a recognition of the importance of the past in terms of ancestors; of the present in terms of the designated group belongingness; and of the future when one becomes oneself an ancestor. There is a pattern of social interactions which I choose to describe as mutual interdependency. Thus, the emphasis in Japan is on a highly structured and vertical society, a promotion of a group sense of identity, and an emphasis on mutual interdependency.

Consideration of therapy for Japanese patients must then include proper responses to these cultural differences. For example, in view of the vertical society, the doctor (Sensei) may have to play the role of an authoritative person. This would make sense in the cultural context. Similarly, the family must often be considered since the identity is a group identity. One's sense of belongingness is an important part of the socialization. This is reflected in Japan, for example, in the practice of having someone from the family stay in the room with the patient in the hospital. The relative's responsibility would be not only to take care of the patient, but to cook and serve the accustomed food for the patient. Although this may be difficult to do in American hospitals, certainly the family can more often be seen to assess what sort of group strengths there are. The parallel in the evaluation of an American patient would be an evaluation of the patient's individual strengths and weaknesses. Just as we do this with individuals in the American culture, so it may be important to evaluate the family, its strengths and weaknesses for a Japanese patient. Finally, therapy may not necessarily be aimed at increasing self-awareness, self-actualization, or individuation. Rather, with the unacculturated Japanese patient, it may be more important to help him to reassume the role of a member of a social group, functioning and contributing towards the welfare of others.

REFERENCES

Butcher, J. N. and Panchari, P.
    1976 A Handbook of Cross-National MMPI Research. University of Minnesota Press, Minneapolis, Minnesota.

Gordon, J. M.
    1964 Assimilation in American Life. Oxford University Press, New York.

Kitano, H. H. L.
    1969 Japanese Americans. Prentice-Hall, Inc., Englewood Cliffs, New Jersy.

Lam, Julia M. D.
    1976 Personal communication.

Lebra, T. S.
    1976 Japanese Pattern of Behavior. The University Press of Hawaii, Honolulu.

Nakane, C.
    1970 Japanese Society. University of California Press, Berkeley and Los Angeles.

Spitzer, R. L., and Endicott, J.,
    1967 and 1968, "DIAGNO" (A Computer Program for Psychiatric Diagnosis Utilizing the Differential Diagnostic Procedure). Archives of General Psychiatry 18, June 1968, Research Division, Washington Heights Community Service, New York State Psychiatric Institute and Biometrics Research, New York State Department of Mental Hygiene, New York.

Spitzer, R. L., Endicott, J., And Cohen, G. M.
    Psychiatric Status Schedule, Evaluation Unit, Biometrics Research, New York State Department of Mental Hygiene, New York State Psychiatric Institute, Department of Psychiatry, Columbia University, New York.

A. L. Th. VERDONK, Ph.D.

THE CHILDREN OF IMMIGRANTS IN THE NETHERLANDS: SOCIAL POSITION AND IMPLIED RISKS FOR MENTAL HEALTH

INTRODUCTION

The focus of this paper is on the children of groups of immigrants in the Netherlands, often referred to as minority groups. They include: Moluccans; people of Surinam and the Antilles; and people of Mediterranean countries from where workers are recruited, such as Turkey, Morocco, Yugoslavia, Tunisia, Spain, Portugal, Greece and Italy. The social position of these children in the Netherlands is one of relative arrears in terms of legal status, access to the labour market, and level of education. This disadvantaged status leads to problems which often manifest in deviant forms of behaviour. The data for this paper come from published sources including scientific, governmental, and other reports, and from interviews with people working in the field of mental health.[1]

Before proceeding into the main topic, some general background information is presented.[2]

The Number of Allochtones

Many people of foreign countries have settled in the Netherlands. They include, circa:
- 300,000 repatriated people from the former Netherlands-Indies;
- 155,000–160,000 people from Surinam and the Antilles;
- 32,000 Moluccans;
- 500,000 from the former colonies;
- 115,000 from European countries within the EEC;
- 180,000 from other Mediterranean countries (worker recruitment countries).

Excluding those repatriated from Indonesia, the Central Bureau of Statistics estimated the numbers of children (0–14 years) without Dutch nationality at about 100,000 in 1976, of which one-half originated from Greece, Yugoslavia, Morocco, Turkey, Spain, Portugal and Tunisia. Approximately 25% of all children of immigrants live in Amsterdam, The Hague and Rotterdam.

1. SOCIAL POSITION OF CHILDREN OF IMMIGRANTS

The social position of immigrant children in the Netherlands is largely determined by such social factors as: their legal status, access to education, the labour market and other institutions, cultural background, prejudices of the host society, and policy on several levels as regards recruitment or immigration in general. These social forces, together, cause great inequality for the second generation. This inequality is so pervasive that it is appropriate to use the term "institutionalized social inequality", which means inequality brought about by institutions in our society like the social, legal, educational and welfare machinery. Institutionalized inequality leads unavoidably towards several forms of deviancy, including problems of mental health.

The following section documents the institutionalized inequality for three groups of children of immigrants: Moluccans, people from Surinam and the Antilles, and children of foreign workers from Mediterranean countries.

A. *Moluccans*

The precise number of Moluccan children in the Netherlands is not known. The following figures are an estimate:
— in 1951, circa 12,000;
— in 1959, circa 18,600;
— in 1978, circa 32,600.

Legal Status

The legal status of Moluccans is well-defined as compared with other foreigners in the Netherlands. They have the same rights and duties as the Dutch citizens with the exception of active and passive franchise and military service. But they are persons without a nationality if they do not choose either the Dutch or the Indonesian citizenship.

Education

The governmental Commission Verwey-Jonker, remarked in 1959 that many Moluccan children pursue continued education, but mainly in advanced primary education and technical or domestic science school. The situation is not so good for them in secondary or higher education. Of note is the fact that the results of the Moluccan pupils in advanced primary education are worse than in the practical, technical or domestic science schools. The Commission looked for the causes in the poverty of language (language arrears) and lack of support in the home milieu. Another negative factor is the overcrowding in areas where Moluccans live, with the consequence of a shortage of quiet study space.

Work

The position of the Moluccans on the labour market has deteriorated since 1968. Particularly worrisome is the unemployment of the youth, where the figure is already two or three times higher than the average unemployment. Reasons are looked for in the higher unemployment figures in regions where Moluccans live

THE CHILDREN OF IMMIGRANTS 51

and less mobility of Moluccan youth because of higher group cohesion. Other reasons are:
— prolonged school attendance, which results in later entry in the labour market; these younger people have to gain more money because they are older, and this lessens the interests of the employing companies;
— many Moluccans do not have a certificate after finishing school;
— prejudice on the part of Dutch employers.

Social-Cultural Policy

The policy of the Dutch government is not accepted by the Moluccan community. The Dutch government wants the full development of the Moluccans within Dutch society: "integration with preservation of one's identity". Moluccans want emancipation as Moluccans. They accuse the government of a policy of assimilation.

The Department of CRM (Culture, Recreation and Social Work) subsidizes 38 Moluccan institutions. Moreover, in 1976, the minister of CRM instituted an Advisory Committee for the well-being of Moluccans (Inspraakorgaan Welzijn Molukkers).

Relations with Autochtones

An investigation in 1972 (IKOR, 1972) demonstrated that Turkish and Moluccan people received the most negative score on the social-distance-scale (Bogardus). Surinamese were the next.

B. *Surinamese and Antillians*

Legal Status

Since the independence of Surinam, December 25, 1975, all people with Surinamese nationality are considered foreigners in the Netherlands. But there are special regulations: they can enter the Netherlands on condition they have means of subsistence and adequate living. Their legal status is comparable with that of people of countries within the European Economic Community. Much depends on the flexibility of Dutch public servants in dealing with alien registration. There are quite a number of complaints over unjust and harsh treatment of foreign people as well as over interpretation and even abnegation of rules and regulations of the treaty between Surinam and the Netherlands (Spannoe, 1978, nr. 4).

Work

Unemployment of Surinamese and Antillian juveniles is very high. Of the age-category of 20–24 years, 20–25% in Amsterdam, The Hague and Rotterdam are without a job.

Since 1974, some special measures have been taken, focussed on several elements. For example:

— improvement of starting position on the labour market by labour habituation, training and education;

— the government has instituted Centers for Professional Orientation and Training. (In May 1975, these centers had 2,400 course-members among whom 200 were Surinamese.)

— the government has tried to improve the mediation for labour by special labour mediators;

— the government has tried to make it attractive for companies to accept Surinamese by a regulation of the costs of wages (an allowance of 30% with a special raise for social provisions).

Housing

Some quarters in Amsterdam and Rotterdam have been "closed" for foreign workers and Surinamese and Antillians. Concentration in old quarters has increased, at least in Rotterdam (Verdonk, 1979). There is a real risk of stigmatization of this physically recognizable group. Moreover, overcrowding in these relatively densely populated areas is rather common for the big families of this minority group which has implications for available study facilities.

Education

Surinamese and Antillian children generally suffer from considerable arrears at school for a number of reasons. One of them is that Dutch is not spoken at home. Furthermore, education in Surinam or the Antillians is of a lower level, or the education systems are different. Dutch education does not fit in with the experience of these children in their home country and at home. In general, the problems of these children are identical with those of Moluccan children. The Ministry of Education and Science has taken some measures:

— the appointment of extra teachers on behalf of reception and accompaniment of these children;

— the Bijlmer project of the Amsterdam Centre of Advice and Accompaniment aimed at designing new education material adjusted to Surinamese children, as well as coaching of teachers who deal with these children;

— attention given to the youth beyond school age, via an experiment in a centre of formation. (In this centre, there is complementary primary education, formation and consultations as regards working.)

Culture

There are many subgroups in the Surinamese population, among others: Creoles, Hindustani, Chinese and Javanese. Cultural adaptation seems much more difficult for the Hindustani than for Creoles because of religion, indigenous customs, and strong accentuation of the family and kinship ties.

Many Surinamese are very conscious too of the colonial relations and the slavery of the past.

Image Held by Autochtones

The image of the Surinamese has deteriorated since 1968–69. At that time, the Autochtone population had a rather propitious idea of Surinamese – the Dutch were mainly friendly, but looked down upon them. Research in 1975 and 1977 showed a negative change. Bovenkerk (1977) demonstrated with tests at the Amsterdam labour market that Surinamese were discriminated against in 22% of 162 cases.

Social-Cultural Activities

There were in 1972, 5 institutions with 27 co-operators; in 1974, 21 institutions with 27 co-operators, in 1978, 24 institutions with circa 350 co-workers, 100% subsidized by the government.

Policy

The policy of the Ministry of Culture, Recreation and Social Work toward Surinamese and Antillians is much the same as with the other minorities: integration with preservation of the proper identity. The policy slogan is now: "participation in society on an equal basis". Nevertheless, there is much criticism of governmental policy by Surinamese social workers on the following lines:

(1) governmental policy is formed without consultation of Surinamese and Antillian immigrants;

(2) governmental policy does not pay enough attention to remigration projects,

(3) there is not enough support and appreciation of Surinamese organizations of welfare work.

Governmental public servants reply that Surinamese organizations reach only a small group of clients and therefore are not representative of the population concerned.

C. *Children of Foreign Workers (Mediterranean)*

Members of families of foreign workers have mainly come to the Netherlands since 1972:

In 1972, 3768 work permits were given to foreigners on account of family reunion; in 1973, 2308; in 1974, 3635.

In the years to come, Turkish and Moroccans in particular will be reuniting with their families here.

Legal Status

The legal status of families of foreign workers is very different from that occupied by Moluccans, Surinamese, and Antillians, and is characterized by inequality, supposition of a temporary stay and dependence. The inequality is a cumulation of juridical inequality and de facto unequal treatment. For example, foreigners have no right to vote. Foreigners often do not satisfy legal regulations to receive benefits. For example, the right to get sickness benefit is connected to the place of residence; this leads to a loss of rights in the case of the foreign worker who goes back to his country.

Supposition of Temporary Stay

The legislation for foreigners implies that a permit to stay here can be refused. In case of unemployment or divorce (both situations wherein one suffers a lack of earnings) and in case of penal offence, there is still a possibility of expulsion. This holds too for the second generation that is, the children. These children only have permission to stay because of familial reunion policies.

Dependence

The public servants have ample power to execute regulations. Many regulations can only be found in circulars which are not published or are difficult to get. This leads to greater dependence on assistants. The weak legal status is a double brake on the process of integration: it causes the feeling of not being accepted in this society; and it influences the readiness to adapt negatively. At the same time, this unequal legal status legitimizes unequal treatment by Dutchmen.

Work

Research confirms that the parents of these immigrant children on the whole are: manual workers, unskilled or at the utmost, half trained; mainly working in secondary segments of the labour market, often in a shift system. There is a sharp distinction in the labour market between skilled and unskilled labour which affects earnings. When the children enter the labour market, they will most probably get the same positions as their fathers (Verdonk, 1979b).

Measures

Neither foreign workers nor their children are considered by officials as groups with arrears — they are only temporarily here. Therefore, there does not exist a governmental policy to improve their position. With regards to juvenile unemployment (Motief, 1979, p. 8) officially there were on December 24, 1978, 1911 juvenile foreigners unemployed. More problems are expected in the future becuase, in the next two years, another 5000 people will leave school and enter the labour market. One expects the employers to be more selective, which is nearly always disadvantageous for members of minority groups. Influencing factors are: lack of a good education; difficulties in speaking and understanding Dutch; lack of a setting which stimulates orientation to Dutch society; and unwillingness of the employers to employ members of cultural minorities.

Education

Relatively few children of immigrants from Mediterranean countries go on to secondary education, as can be seen from the following table:

	Infant Class Primary School[a]		Secondary School (VWO–MAVO–HAVO)[b]		Lower Technical School[b]	
	Pupils from 7 Recruitment-Countries + Italy	Other Countries	Pupils from 7 Recruitment-Countries + Italy	Other Countries	Pupils from 7 Recruitment-Countries + Italy	Other Countries
1975	14.329	5.357	1.549	2.169	1.448	389
1976	17.456	6.293	2.049	3.041	?	?
1977	20.511	7.086	2.528	3.584	?	?

Sources: CBS, Hoofdafdeling Statistieken van Onderwijs en Wetenschappen.
[a] January 16
[b] September 1
Wetenschappelijke Raad voor het Regeringsbeleid, 1979, p. 140.

The report of a conference on the second generation (Stichting Welzijn Buitenlandse Werknemers Oost-Brabant, 1979) states that:

— there are scarcely any educational provisions for children 16 and older;
— children attend school classes which do not correspond with their level of intelligence;
— some children of 12–13 years of age do not attend school at all;
— many children are behind in school;
— not enough opportunities for illiterates;
— The International Connection Class (Internationale Schakelklas) should not be linked only with Lower Technical Schools but also with other schools for secondary education.

Factors influencing the educational problems of foreign children are:
— Dutch is not their native language;
— they do not get enough support of their parents because these people do not understand the Dutch education system;
— contacts between parents and school are scarce;
— ideas and norms of parents are often conflicting with the ones of schools;
— motivation to study Dutch is sometimes low because some still hope one day to return to the home country (Verdonk, 1979b.)

Categorical Welfare Work

The ministry of Culture, Recreation and Social Work completely subsidizes 18 regional institutions. Moreover, the Netherlands Centrum voor Foreigners has an overarching role as a consulting partner with the Ministry and gives service to refugees and people asking for asylum. There are a number of tensions. The Ministry of CRM has no influence in decisions to attract foreign workers for the labour market (which is mainly determined by economic criteria). The CRM has to cope with the social consequences of a policy, made by others. Welfare workers are in a fierce debate about integration or emancipation and categorical versus general approaches.

Clubs/Associations

Some self-organization is growing among the foreign workers' groups to promote their own interests and those of the children. Some youth clubs have been organized together with political organizations. The churches too have taken initiatives on behalf of the foreign population.

Attitude of Dutch to Foreigners

— the score on the "social distance scale" is rather negative for the Turk, the Moroccan and the Spaniard when compared with other ethic groups;
— in case of a criminal offence, the nationality of the offender is mentioned too often in the papers;
— research of Bovenkerk (1977) showed that Amsterdam employers discriminated against the Spanish as well as the Surinamese.

Policy on Institutional Level

The principles of policy for attracting foreign workers have remained relatively unchanged:
— guest workers are here temporarily; they function as a temporary conjuncture buffer, coming in at the moment of an upward movement in the labour market and going out at the moment of decline;

— the necessity to employ foreign workers is still there and will continue.
— the Netherlands is not a country of immigration although there are differing opinions on that issue at high levels of the ministries.

Cultural Differences

The second generation of immigrants is educated in a Dutch system of values and norms, which can bring conflicts with the parents. This is especially true for cultures which differ greatly from the Dutch (like Hindustan, Turkish, Moroccan, Tunisian). The following report (Marzak, 1979) on a Moroccan family illustrates such value conflicts:

In Morocco, the father remains at a distance to maintain his authority. The son has to kiss his father's hand when the latter comes home and then has to sit back or leave the room. Sexuality is taboo. If the son wants to marry, he talks with his mother.

Life of youth in the Netherlands is much more free. Youth may go with girlfriends and boyfriends and choose their own clothes. In this situation, if a Moroccan father nevertheless asks for strict obedience and the child disagrees, contact between father and son will be scarce.

Mother brings the children up until they are 8 years old. After that age, the girls continue to be with the mother. The boys go out to participate in the world of the men and they are not in the home. Sons and daughters must obey their parents. If not, they do not give honour to their parents, and may get a sound drubbing. The girl has to obey all men in the home, even to the younger brothers, and to the older woman in the house. She has to be chaste; if not, she brings shame and infamy to the family. The girl has to look after the younger children. She goes normally to the domestic science school because there it is good preparation for matrimony, and she will not meet boys.

Honour- and infamy-complex is central in Moroccan culture. Nobody can behave without honour because this has effects for the whole group. The loss of honour asks for reaction, and sometimes a violent one. Public opinion defines the status of the group; this eventually leads to preserving some appearance. The "show outside" seems more important than "truth inside".

The Dutch are criticized because of the relations between man and woman, and parents and children. The Moroccan often thinks that the Dutch woman is the boss in the home and that she has ample sexual liberty. Thus the Dutch husband has no honour. A Dutch child of 18 years does what he likes, and does not give respect. Parents and children treat each other as equals. This creates anguish in the Moroccan.

The Dutch wonder why the Moroccan woman seems so dependent. When friends come visiting, the woman has to leave the room or at least be silent. Women and children are beaten and locked in, according to the stereotyped image in Holland.

The above example gives some aspects of Moroccan culture. Other societies have their own unique customs. Children often have conflicts because they live in two cultures. Case studies (Soetens, 1978) give excellent examples. It is absolutely necessary for the social assistant to know the culture of different cultural groups very well in order to give adequate help.

Conclusion

The social position of children of ethnic minorities is defined by a number of social elements. These include:
— a weak legal status; this holds more for the children of immigrant workers than for Moluccans, Surinamese and Antillians. Moreover, the legal status is not identical with the socially determined possibilities to execute one's rights;
— a parental milieu in which the father has normally a low socio-economic position;
— a good chance to get behind at school because of poverty of language, few stimuli from the parental milieu, and uncertainty as to when one will return to the home country;
— a stereotyped approach by Autochtones, which often leads to exclusion from the labour market,
— living in the Dutch culture which often leads to conflicts with parents;
— welfare institutions which only recently became conscious of these problems;
— the unequal treatment of minority groups by the Dutch government;
— governmental policy that guest workers are going to stay only temporarily, which discourages any effort to do anything about the underprivileged position of the children of foreign workers;
— the gap between integration on an institutional level — the level of governmentally subsidized or created institutions and self-organizations, and integration at the level of personal contacts, that is, discrimination is forbidden by law but occurs in fact.

Social position is the place one gets in society — assigned or chosen by oneself — by the interplay of the above-mentioned social forces. These forces limit freedom of movement and possibilities of rising in society. They affect self-respect, self-realization, or realization of an entire group. They fence the person in; they keep him within social bounds.

Not every immigrant is affected by the same combination of social circumstances. For example, the Moluccans are distinguished from other ethnic minority groups by their political aspirations. However, the curtailment by social circumstances more often than not evokes reactions which other parts of society label as deviancy. The social limitations are such that these reactions are socially predictable and will occur, time and again. A number of these reactions will be described in the second part of this paper.

2. PROBLEMATIC REACTIONS OF CHILDREN OF MINORITIES

Some immigrant children manifest behaviour reactions such as mental disorders, use of drugs, running away from home, aggression and apathy. Scientific research in this field is virtually absent in the Netherlands. For this paper, we draw from reports of several institutions which are concerned, as well as from interviews.[3]

A. *Moluccans*

The relationship between Moluccans and Dutchmen is affected by violence and scuffles occurring in the late 1960s. Experts are divided over the causes. Political as well as social motives play a role. According to Marien (1971), the following factors have an influence on the repeated expressions of violence among the Moluccan youth:[7]

− sources of discomfort within the Moluccan community as, for example, alienation between parents and children;

− discomfort because of failing social emancipation characterized by poverty of language and by prejudice and discrimination on the part of the Dutch society, particularly on the labour market;

− the Moluccans have a special demographic structure, with many young people born in the Netherlands, who left school institutions in 1966.

The social position of Moluccans is weaker now. One observes an increase in usage of hard drugs, and in the number of young people fighting for their ideal of a free Moluccan Republic. Moluccan drug users are mostly young people, disillusioned in their ideals, who cannot realize themselves in Duth society. They have no horizon and do not see possibilities for the future. It is questionable if social accompaniment in the normal sense has a solution for this problem.

B. *Surinamese and Antillians*

According to Ramlal,[4] the awareness of colonial exploitation has effects on one's psychic make-up in the following three ways:

− in the colonial period, man is dehumanized to keep going the production process. As a consequence of this colonial relation, the Surinamese behave like white men in order to be recognized as human beings;

− in relation to this colonial complex, we see dependent behaviour towards the Dutchman;

− a marginal existence is maintained; one continues to carry the expectation of returning to Surinam.

Thus, the Surinamese identify with Dutchmen and reject them at the same time.

Another problem is the high rate of divorce. In Surinam, the woman was very dependent on her husband. The freedom in Holland means a rise in status for her, and corresponding loss of status for the man. Some 25% of all Hindustani families in The Hague are divorced (1500 families). One can only make conjectures about the consequence for the children because of the difficult situation at home. The children often get into trouble at school. They start complaining, and run away.

Quite a number of these children enter into special schools because of study or behavioural problems.

In the big cities, one is confronted now with the so-called "hossel" culture among unemployed juvenile Surinamese, with elements of violence, criminality and drug abuse. This is particularly the case among the unskilled, young people in the lowest strata who express behaviour characterized by hardness, aggressiveness, and a rejection of all behaviour of whites.

In 1977, a report of ICBM (Problematic Drug Use, 1977) states that the number of drug abusers has risen sharply among younger Surinamese. At an estimate, they form 20% of all drug users in the Netherlands with circa 2000 of the addicted concentrated in the big cities. Assistance will be effective only if circumstances which lead to this drug abuse are changed; for example, if Dutch society offers real possibilities for good housing, employment and professional training. Another report of ICBM (1978) observes again the insufficiency of the existing policy.

Other problems are mentioned too, such as alcoholism, gambling, and a relative high number of unmarried mothers (Concept Policy Report, Mental Health Care Rotterdam, 1977). Finally, a research by Hettinga (1978) in a psychiatric institution (Santpoort, where 51 Surinamese patients were admitted) mentions some important circumstances in relation to psychiatric admission:

— unemployment or bad circumstances at work (13 patients);

— housing (13 patients),

— alcohol and drug abuse (14 patients);

— relational problems (22 patients);

— generational problems (2 patients, traditional relations of authority in the family were broken up);

— adaptation problems (8 patients; ambivalence in returning to Surinam);

— identity problems (many patients are in doubt over their identity: are they Creole, Hindustan, Surinamese, Dutch?); the identity problems had also to do with sexual identity.

This research gives a good idea of the problems of Surinamese psychiatric patients. In addition to psychiatric breakdown, other forms of problem behaviour are found such as youths running away from home. For example, an interview with the Office for Tracing Children in Rotterdam revealed that Surinamese children run away more often than all other groups. A number of them go back home; others are referred to Pro Juventute, Psychic Social Work, Council of Juvenile Protection. Finally, there is the matter of abortion. Figures of Stimezo demonstrated that in 1978, 10% of all abortions in the age category of 10–24 years involved Surinamese women (about 500 cases). Ketting[5] considers the percentage of Surinamese women rather high because the age category in the entire Dutch population is lower than 10%. Exact statistics on the number of Surinamese women in this age category are lacking. It is known that most of these women are unmarried at the time of abortion, that 65% of the Surinamese had no children, and that 18% of Surinamese had already had an earlier abortion.

C. *Children of Mediterranean Immigrants*

Epidemiological data are not available for this group. Problems indicated by health workers are the following:

— study problems;

— different value and normsystems at home and in the school;

— insecurity due to uncertainty about the family's return to the home country, which leads to difficulties in emotional attachment and to identity conflicts;

— great dependence on parents, especially in Turkish and Moroccan families;

— intensification of generation conflicts, because the children do better in the Dutch society and thus menace the authoritative relations in the family;

— parents, confronted with problems of their children (insolence, stealing, not studying etc.), lock themselves in their own culture.

In considering the provision of help to these children, one must be aware of the honor and shame complex. It is a disgrace when problems are brought to others. That is one of the reasons why an assistant has difficulty gaining access to the family. If one starts a therapeutic program for children, one needs permission of the parents. Which standpoint have we to take? In many families, the woman is completely dependent on the husband. It is suspicious when a woman has to make contact with a male assistant. Moroccan and Turkish women are very difficult to contact, and yet, they have the responsibility of looking after the young children.

There seems to be a difference in the problems of boys and girls. Boys show more difficulties at school; or at least the parents think that; and via the general practitioner, they are referred to social psychiatric services. Girls go to Youth Advice Centres and show more behavioural difficulties. These data are confirmed by the observations of the Rotterdam Municipal Working Group Health Care migrants (1979). At this moment, there are only a few drug addicted (circa 10 Turkish and 30 North Africans). However, assistants fear there is a potential group of addicts found in the children of the second generation of immigrants.

Usage of Institutions of Mental Health Care

The Rotterdam Nota of Migranten (1978) observes that immigrants from the Mediterranean countries make little use of mental health facilities, as shown in the Table I:

TABLE I

Total Number of patients and migrants in care of or referred by the Department of Social Psychiatry and Mental Hygiene of G. G. and G. D.

	Migrants	Total
In care of neighbourhood Teams (1−2−1978)	36	1661
Children in home, in care of SPGH (1−2−1978)	0	170
In care of the subdepartment alcohol and drugs	5	103
Referred to psychiatric institutions (1977)	48	1410
In care of halfway-institutions (homes etc.)	0	160
In psychotherapy (1−2−1978)	0	70

Source: Nota Migranten Rotterdam 1978, Bijlage 16. (Report Migrants in Rotterdam, 1978, appendix 16)

In Rotterdam, there are no children placed in a home because of psycho-therapeutic reasons. Immigrants in care of neighbourhood teams or psychiatric institutions are underrepresented. Only 119 per 100,000 immigrants were in care of neighbourhood teams versus 290 per 100,000 of the whole Rotterdam population; and 158 per 100,000 immigrants were admitted to psychiatric institutions versus 243 per 100,000 of the whole Rotterdam population. Immigrant children are underrepresented too in the Foundation of Mental Health Care of Rotterdam. About 10% of 750 cases referred per year to one of the organizations (MOB, LMSPD) are Surinamese, Antillian or Mediterranean, but only very few continue psychotherapeutic treatment.

Runaways (Children Traced by the Police)

Systematic data on runaway children of immigrants in the Netherlands are lacking.[6] There are some figures in Rotterdam, given by the police head of the Children's Department. In 1978, there were 183 children of immigrant who were missed and had to be traced. Surinamese, Turkish and Moroccan children are most numerous. About 10% of the total runaway population (0−19 years) in 1978 belonged to the Mediterranean countries. Many of the children traced by the police are referred to the following: the Council of Youth Protection, the Medical Educational Office, JAC (Youth Advice Centre), the GG and GD (Municipal Health Department), the Foundation Welfare Work for Surinamese, and Psycho-Social Work. According to the police, the following types of situations characterize the backgrounds of the runaway children; Turkish boys reject the absolute way of authority of their father, the girls do not want to be given in marriage. This holds too for Moroccan and Hindustani girls. Turkish and

Moroccan boys are sometimes beaten up. Spanish and Portuguese children, accustomed to severe authority, experience much freedom here. These children get confused in two norm-systems, and do not know what to do anymore. Are there typical criminal offences carried out by foreign youth? Generally not, but male prostitution occurs among Moroccans and some foreign girls are involved in prostitution. The police estimates that in Rotterdam about 50 Dutch and foreign girls of 15 years of age give services for payment. The number of girls of 18 years and older who function this way is unknown. There is the impression that foreign children steal a bit more from big department stores than do their Dutch counterparts. A case in point is a Turkish girl, celebrating her 13th birthday, who was taken to the police station because she had stolen 2 cassette recorder tapes. It turned out that her parents had given her a cassette recorder for her birthday but no tapes. There does not seem to be any organized criminal youth gangs. In conclusion, it seems that the proportion of foreign children running away is not very much larger than the Dutch counterparts, but exact figures are lacking.

Abortion

Because of a lack of comparable figures, it is not possible to say if foreign Mediterranean women have more abortions than do Dutch or Surinamese women. Available statistics indicate that 50% of the Mediterranean women having an abortion were married, versus circa 20% in the other two groups. A greater number of Surinamese and Mediterranean women have had an abortion before, as compared with other groups.

Conclusions

Exact data about psychological complaints and the use of institutions of mental health care by immigrants are lacking in the Netherlands. Health workers have the impression that psychic problems among the immigrant populations are multiple and difficult to handle because of differences in culture. The prevalent problems concern study problems of boys, behavioural difficulties of girls, and conflicts between parents and children. On the whole, a considerable number of children have arrears at school. The number of Mediterranean children running away from home does not seem much higher than that of Dutch, although there are no exact figures. There are indications that mental health institutions are less used by immigrants than by Dutch people.

3. THEORIES ABOUT PSYCHOLOGICAL PROBLEMS

A theory tries to explain why a phenomenon occurs via a series of interconnected concepts. If one understands why a phenomenon occurs, it is possible to take action. In the section which follows, the phenomena described in Part Two are explained according to various authors with a psychological, cultural, anthropological or sociological paradigm (Verdonk, 1977).

A. *Psychological Paradigm*

At least 2 variants can be described. In the first, one tries to understand psychological problems via the concept of internalization of the judgement of the dominant majority. Reactions of people may be different: they start behaving according to the concept of the majority and one can speak of a self-fulfilling prophecy. Or one turns completely to the culture of the dominant majority, such as wishing to be white. A third reaction may be the rejection of the stereotype, with something akin to the Black Power Movement (for example, each Dutchman is a colonial and should be fought until the bitter end). We may perhaps understand the "hossel culture" with this concept.

The second variant is the concept of identity conflict: above all, tensions within the person get attention (i.e. tensions originated by his life within two cultures). One does not know anymore who one is: Surinamese, Hindustani, Dutchman? As a reaction, it is possible that the person no longer is able to have emotional attachments (Kabela, 1974).

B. *Cultural-Anthropological Paradigm*

The "base personality" formed in the first years of childhood comes in conflict with values and norms from another culture, which has been internalized especially by the second generation. Also, there exist acculturation problems: difficulties in adapting to a new strange culture. There is an "allergia entre des structures psychologiques et interiorisés à partir des symboliques socio-culturelles de milieu d'origine et du milieu d'accueil", (De Almeida, 1971). One supposes that children of the second generation are, at the same time, attached to old standards and models of behaviour while confronted with the necessity to adopt new values and norms.

C. *Sociological Paradigm*

There are several variants here. One is that problems are caused by different acculturation of parents and children in the new culture. Parents cling to old traditional values and norms and accept parts of the Dutch culture. For example, a Spanish father says to his daughter who invites friends home: "no boyfriends unless he is your 'novio', and once married, always married." At the same time, he says that he likes to stay in Holland, and animates his children to study well and to participate in Dutch sports life.

He does not make contacts with Spanish people but refuses to make contacts with the Dutch.

Another hypothesis is that of "goal striving stress" (Parker, Kleiner, 1969).

Children have to work hard, but cannot cope with their significant models. The ambition of the parents plays a role in the pressures on the child. There is social disorganization if the authority and influence of an earlier culture and system of social control is undermined and eventually destroyed (Park, 1959). Social disorganization leads to personal disorganization in which a person cannot function effectively because he lives with contradictory standards of behaviour, which causes inner confusion.

Merton might speak of his several types of reaction on a socially predefined situation. In many societies, anomie exists as a consequence of the gap between the culturally and socially defined aims and the social limited means to reach these aims. Reactions, as described in Part Two, may be described along the lines of his four types of reactions: *the innovator, the ritualist, the rejector* and *the rebel* (Verdonk, 1979a). Penninx (Rapport, WRR, 1979; Penninx) mentions the theory of unequal chances to explain the social backward position of minority groups. In this theory, one supposes that it is in principle possible to create equal chances for everybody. This seems to be questionable, surely, for those minorities for whom the economic motive is the main reason to attract them to Holland.

To my mind, the *institutionalized social inequality* is probably the root too of problems as described in Part Two. In Part One of the paper, we have seen that there exists great inequality on the level of institutions, like the legal status, education, entry in the labour market, political and cultural participation. This inequality is the resultant of social forces which are embodied in these institutions. The result is that it is virtually impossible for the children of minority groups to break through these social fences. This is at the root of the reactions of a number of young people. They are not blind to the social problem of inequality nor to the social resistance to their emancipation battle to win self-respect, prestige, income and a social position. Their reactions will differ. There are some who individualize the problem of social inequality; say that they are not capable enough to get over the threshold, get disheartened, eventually get depressed. Others consider it impossible to fight against this enormous, untouchable social colossus which is our institutionalized society. They may fly away in a dream world of dance, in apathy, in narrowminded individualism, in the drug scene, in a dream of the original country as "paradise lost", or in psychic problems.

Another category recognizes the problem and tries to gain a social position for themselves by working very hard. They try to conquer the social machinery individually. The price is often that the social fabric continues although it offers a better position to an individual member. I am reminded then of a free bird in a golden cage. Finally, we see people who try to fight against social inequality via collective actions in a battle for emancipation. There will come initiatives to improve the legal status, to create possibilities for professional training, to ameliorate working conditions, to fight against racism and discrimination. These reactions are brought forward by the awareness of institutionalized inequality.

These reactions are social definitions of the minority-majority-situation and, as such, are not exclusively individual responses on a social question.

I think that this hypothesis gives a reasonable explanation of a number of drop-outs among children of ethnic minorities. Clearly this is an option. The stress hypothesis, personal disorganization as consequence of social disorganization, difference in phase of acculturation, cultural differences and conflicts offer a partial explanation; the theory of deviancy as a socially defined and determined reaction on institutionalized social inequality is broader and may incorporate these other hypotheses. One can even think that specific problems which are explainable with the hypotheses of goal-striving stress are deducible from this social inequality. Thus, we create a hierarchy of hypotheses which may explain the social production of deviancy.

4. POSSIBILITIES FOR PREVENTION

Preventive action should direct efforts to the educational institution, the labour market, image building of Autochtones and Allochtones, governmental policy etc. These actions, though primary preventive (Caplan, 1964), do not belong normally to the mental health care worker. Social workers, action groups, self-organizations of foreigners, syndicates, governmental bodies, and churches have a task here. However, mental health care should have this background knowledge as a framework for its own actions.

But there are other needs too. They include:

— service provided by functionaries who really know something of the culture and customs of the home country, and have therapeutic expertise to help people with problems, or at least can give consultations;

— an example is given by a project for Surinamese mothers in The Hague. (The Dutch model of assistance is not adequate; Surinamese mothers do not come when they get a written invitation to talk. There has to be a clear offer; e.g. we are going to talk two hours on ways to spend your money, education of children, drugs, etc.).

— stimulation of youth projects, where a good combination exists of pleasant and useful things; these groups can talk about difficulties at home, relations with boys and girls, Autochtones and Allochtones, drugs, etc.

— securing more precise and scientific information about the number of youth with mental health problems, as well as their participation rate in mental health institutions.

Apart from that, we should analyze case studies of people referred to institutions like Social Psychiatric Services, Psychic Social Work Council of Juvenile Protection etc., to learn if there are patterns in the problems and to do something with it. Furthermore, theories should be developed more extensively to understand better how the social machinery of our society creates strains which force people to turn to some form of deviancy.

NOTES

[1] I wish to thank Alet van 't Eind who helped me in preparing this paper. There was a group interview with health workers from several cities in the Netherlands, as well as with Drs Ramlal, Director of the Foundation for Surinamers in The Hague, Inspector van Oudheusden and Mrs Steinmetz, Department of the Vice Squad and Children's Police, Rotterdam. Drs T. van der Grinten, Director of the Netherlands Centre for Mental Health (NCGV), organized the above mentioned group discussion together with Mr C. Blankestijn, Advisor of the Netherlands Association for Ambulant Mental Health Care (NVAGG). Acknowledgements too to Mr Ketting of NISSO for making available data on abortion; to Mr Khargie, member of ICBM (Interdepartmental Commission for Coordination of Policy on behalf of Migrants from Surinam and the Dutch Antilles) working at CBUVR (Central Office for Implementation of Housing Policy for Citizins of Surinam and the Dutch Antilles).

[2] This general information comes largely from a very recently published report of a governmental commission, namely Report WRR Etnische Minderheden, finished May 9, 1979 and published in June 1979. This information confirms the findings and impressions which I gathered in 1978. For Dutch-reading students see Verdonk, 1979b.

[3] Alet van 't Eind has been asked to look for some North American literature which dealt with second generation immigrants, especially in relation to mental health. And if so, if solutions for mental health problems are reported. She has looked for answers in the following books:

Dollard, J.
    1937 Caste and Class in Southerntown. Harper & Brothers, New York.
Dollard, J. and A. Davis
    1940 Children of Bondage, American Council on Education, Washington, D. C.
Strong, E. K.
    1934 The Second Generation Japanese Problem. Stanford University Press, Stanford University.
Handlin, O.
    1966 Children of the Uprooted. George Brazilles, New York.
Kessner, T.
    1977 The Golden Door, Italian and Jewish Immigrants' Mobility in New York City 1880–1915. Oxford University Press.
Brody, E.
    1968 Minority Groups' Adolescents in the United States M.D.

This literature is written or influenced by the period of the Chicago school; more or less anthropological descriptions of cities and communities, where immigrants live and work. These studies are very descriptive, more of the quality of a good television documentary film. Much is said about cultural values. Nothing is said about solutions for the problems of the second generation, with the exception of the Japanese.

Strong (o. c., 1937) points to a number of social and economic conditions to solve the problems of the Japanese second generation: information about US professions, and choices of professions and actions to provide work.

This lack of provisions and solutions seems influenced by the fact that ethic minorities had the chance to form their own communities. Thus their identity is largely determined by their own culture.

[4] Ramlal: personal communication.

[5] Ketting, cooperator of NISSO (Netherlands Institute of Social Sexuological Research) has given data of all policlinics which are linked with STIMEZO (Foundation of Medical Breaking of Pregnancy). Circa 1/3 or 1/25 of all abortions occur in hospitals; these data are not in this list.

[6] According to a personal communication of Mr. van Oers, Member of the Governmental Coordination Commission for Scientific Research Child Protection (Coordinatie Commissie Wetenschappelijk Onderzoek Kinderbescherming) there are no reliable estimations of the number of children of ethnic minorities who ran away from home.

Recently the commission has decided not to start an investigation because the group of potential children running away is thought to be too small.

[7] Research mentioned in the text and not in the list of literature is cited from Report WRR 1979.

REFERENCES

Almeida, Z. de et al.
　1970　Difficultés d'integration dans les grandes villes rureaux et étrangers, Table Ronde. La Santé Mentale, No. 1, Nov. 28.
Alofs, B. en Bruinessen van M. Turkije
　1977　N. C. B. I. S. M. N. O. I. V. B. Dec.
Autrement
　1977　Culture immigree, No. 11, November.
Bagley, C.
　1968　Migration race and mental health; A review of some recent research in Race IX, 3.
Berthelier, R.
　1977　Hygiène mentale de l'adolescent migrant. Comité Medical et Medico-Social d'aide aux Migrants, April: 13–17.
Bovenkerk, F.
　1977　Rasdiscriminatie op de Amsterdamse Arbeidsmarkt (Race-discrimination on the labour market of Amsterdam) Sociologische Gids XX IV: 58–60.
Bureau Voorlichting Gezondheidszorg Buitenlanders
　1978–79　Literatuurlijst: Voorlichting Gezondheidszorg Buitenlanders. Postbus 3200, 3502 GE Utrecht. (Information Office Health Care for Foreigners. List of Literature: Information on Health Care for Foreigners.)
Caplan, G.
　1964　Principles of Preventive Psychiatry. London, Tavistock.
Coenen, W.
　1978　Jeugdwerkloosheid (Youth-unemployment). Motief 5, p. 8.
Concept Beleidsnota Geestelijke Gezondheidszorg
　1977　Gemeente Rotterdam, Secretarie afdeling Sociale Zaken Volksgezondheid en Wijkaangelegenheden. Het kind in tel. 1979 Centraal Bureau voor Statistiek, Den Haag. (Concept Policy Report Mental Health Care Town of Rotterdam, Secretary Social Affairs, Public Health and Matters of Districts, Children counted.)
Hettinga, N.
　1978　Surinaamse psychiatrische patiënten in Nederland. Scriptie Sociale Psychiatrie, Nijmegen, October. (Surinamese psychiatric patients in the Netherlands. Essay in Social Psychiatry, Nijmegen, October.)
Interdepartementale Commissie voor Beleidscoordinatie ten behoeve van Migranten uit Suriname en de Nederlandse Antillen (ICBM)
　1978　Nota jeugdige Surinaamse migranten in Nederland. Maart. (Interdepartmental Commission for Coordination of Policy on behalf of Migrants from Suriname and the Dutch Antilles. Report on young Surinamese migrants in the Netherlands. March.)
Jeugdwerkloosheid, Tweede Kamer der Staten Generaal, Zitting, 1978–79: No. 15: 541. (Youth unemployment, Second Chamber of States-General, Session 1978–79, No. 15: 541.)

Kabela, M.
1973 Het kind van de rekening, Een Sociaal-Psychologische beschrijving van de aanpassingsproblematiek van kinderen van Spaanse buitenlandse werknemers, in Tijdschrift voor Maatschappelijke Vraagstukken en Welzijnswerk, (19). (Children who have to foot the bill, A social Psychological description of the adaptation problems of children of Spanish workers in Tijdschrift voor Maatschappelijke Vraagstukken en Welzijnswerk, (19).)

Kabela, M.
1974 Kinderen van Spaanse gastarbeiders. M. G. V. 6(29): 296–305. (Children of Spanish workers. M. G. V. 6(29): 296–305.)

Kok, H.
1979 Klub-en buurthuizen ontdekken buitenlanders. Motief 5: 12–13. (Clubs and neighbourhood houses discover foreigners. Motief 5: 12–13.)

Marzak, R.
1978–79 Ik kan en mag er niet om heen. Het probleem van de Marokkaanse kinderen 2e generatie in Helmond. (I cannot and shall not avoid the problem. The problem of Morroccan children of the second generation in Helmond. Katholieke Sociale Academie 'Den Elzent'. Eindhoven, studierichting Maatschappelijk Werk.)

Meer, Ph. van der, Wierx, R. and Spanje, N. C. B.
1977 Utrecht, Postbus 13313, Utrecht.

Mesman Schultz, K. and Methorst, P.
1976 Buitenlandse gedetineerden in Nederland. Wetenschappelijk Onderzoek en Dokumentatie-centrum, Ministerie van Justitie, Den Haag, Maart. (Foreign prisoners in the Netherlands, Scientific Research and Documentation Centre.)

1978 Nota Migranten in Rotterdam, verzameling, S. Z. nr. 22145 (Report on Migrants in Rotterdam, collection.)

Park, R.
1952 Human communities, In: The City and Human Ecology. The Free Press, New York.

Parker, S., Kleiner, R., and Needelman, B.
1969 Migration and mental illness. Some reconsiderations and suggestions for further research. Soc. Science and Medicine 3: 1–9.

Regionale Raad voor de Arbeidsmarkt voor de provincie Zuid-Holland
1979 Nota inzake de werkloosheid onder buitenlandse arbeiders. Rotterdam, Meent 220, April. (Regional Council for the Labour Market of the Province of South Holland. Report of unemployment among foreign workers.)

Rockwell, B.
1979 Jongeren leggen nog aarzelend kontakten. Motief 5: 10–11. (Youth makes hesitating contact. Motief 5: 10–11.)

Soetens, N.
1978 Gastarbeiders, Hun Vrouwen, Hun kinderen. Futile, Rotterdam, 2e druk. (Guestworkers, Their Wives, Their Children, Futile, Rotterdam, second edition.)

Stichting Geestelijke Gezondheidszorg Rotterdam
Projektvoorstel in de vorm van een brief aan de Minister van Cultuur, Recreatie en Maatschappelijk Werk, Steenvoordelaan 370, 2284 CP Rijswijk. (Foundation of Mental Health Care in Rotterdam, Proposal for a Project. Letter to the Ministry of Culture, Recreation and Social Work.)

Stichting Welzijn Buitenlandse Werknemers Oost-Brabant
1979 Verslag Studiedag Tweede Generatie op 3 juni 1978. Eindhoven, January (not published). (Foundation for the Wellbeing of Foreign Workers, East Brabant. Report of the Symposium on the Second Generation, June 3, 1978.)

Tweede Kamer der Staten-General
    1977–78 Nota de problematiek van de Molukse minderheid in Nederland. Zitting No. 14915. (Second Chamber of the States General. Report on the problems of the Moluccan minority in the Netherlands. Session No. 14915.)
Verdonk, A.
    1977 Migration and mental illness. Migration News, No. 4: 9–18.
Verdonk, A.
    1979 (a) Stadsbuurten: De Ene Is de Andere Niet. Relaties tussen psychiatrische opname, andere categorieën van deviantie en kenmerken van gebieden: een sociologische studie. Van Loghum Slaterus, Deventer. (City Areas and Categories of Deviants.)
Verdonk, A.
    1979 (b) Van Gastarbeiders tot immigranten. De problemen van de tweede generatie. M. G. V. 6/7: 444–458. (From guestworkers to immigrants. Problems of the second generation.)
Verveen-Keulemans, F. M.
    1979 Buitenlandse kinderen in de jeugdgezondheidszorg. Tijdschrift voor Soc. Geneeskund 57: 21–29. (Foreign children in health care for young people, Tijdschrift voor Sociale Geneeskund 57: 21–29.)
Werkgroep Gezondheidszorg Migranten Rotterdam
    1979 Tussentijds Verslag. Secretarie Afdeling Sociale Zaken Volksgezondheid en Wijkaangelegenheden. (Work Group on Health Care for Migrants, Rotterdam. Intermediate Report.)
Wetenschappelijke Raad voor het Regeringsbeleid
    1979 Rapporten aan de Regering: Etnische minderheden. Staatsuitgeverij Den Haag. (Scientific Council for Governmental Policy. Reports to the Government: Ethnic minorities. State Publishing House, The Hague.)

BRITT-INGRID STOCKFELT-HOATSON, Ph.D.

EDUCATION AND SOCIALISATION OF MIGRANTS' CHILDREN IN SWEDEN WITH SPECIAL REFERENCE TO BILINGUALISM AND BICULTURALISM*

In this paper, bilingualism and biculturalism will be treated from the viewpoint that these must be the aim of education since the migrants' children must be able to understand both their country of origin and the host country. Many of them will face re-migration, and this should be considered by the school in the host country. The concept of bilingualism may be seen as a sub-concept of biculturalism, because one can hardly conceive of a non-speaking, human society. The word "bilingualism" will here refer to the total mode of communication between human beings, i.e., through verbal as well as non-verbal means such as gestures, airs, and odd sounds like clicks, etc.

Bilingualism is by no means a simple concept. It may be seen as ranging from a capacity to use either of two languages without apparent difficulty to complete command of two languages, so-called "bilingual balance". It is, of course, more common that the bilingual has one language that he prefers, or that he prefers for special purposes. There is a difference between co-ordinate bilingualism, where a person has learned two languages in separate contexts, and compound bilingualism, where one language is learned through the other. Both versions can be more or less functional depending on how favourable the learning situation has been during the individual's formative years.

Co-ordinate or well developed bilingualism, then, will be the result of an adequate linguistic education of immigrant children. A less than adequate education, which is the most common case in most parts of the world may, however, result in an adult who is unable to make sufficient use of either his first or his second language. A compound bilingualism may also be beyond the scope of such a person, at least as a normal school achievement, because he gets the instructions in a language that he does not master.

The deficiencies of inadequate language learning will often be accompanied by a cultural shock to the whole emigrating family. The first language deteriorates, the second is for a long time — perhaps forever — insufficient, and the members of the family experience plain misery. They cannot explain themselves nor their thoughts and emotions in a nuanced manner.

A very common mistake is the underestimating of problems of emigrants from countries where the language resembles the language of the new country, or where some kind of dialect or deviant version is spoken. In Sweden, for example, a great many Norwegian and Danish children are regarded as being in no need of special attention. But they have problems, as do many children from the Swedish-speaking parts of Finland and from the areas along the Finnish border. These children may understand Swedish but have gaps of a linguistic as well as a more general cultural kind which make life hard to understand. They also need guidance into their new country, although this may only require such things as orientation, comparative studies, time for discussion, and so on. Being the teacher of immigrant children is probably one of the most difficult and demanding tasks in a school system. The teacher must know, and understand, the problems of the children, including both problems that are related to the cultural shock as well as problems that relate to the use of differing languages. There are different grammatical difficulties for every linguistic group. Finnish, for example, does not use prepositions as a means to explain direction, position, etc., but has a very intricate system of suffixes and postpositions. There is no difference between "she" and "he" and so on. If the teacher knows about the differences, she/he will be able to explain and understand why some pupils find it hard to learn. It takes a good deal of studies to realize that one's own way of thinking is not the only one. Teachers must also not be deceived by the flow of language that is often produced which gives an impression that the children are much more advanced than they really are. This apparent "understanding" may lead the teacher to continue too fast, and overlook lexical, grammatical, and syntactical deficiencies in both languages. Still worse, the teacher may not realize that the flow is built on very shallow knowledge where many basic concepts are missing. It is absolutely necessary that the teachers learn about the normal acquisition of language and that they have time and instruments for evaluating the immigrant children's progress. The teacher must also be aware that language is not simply transferred from adult to child, but is part of a social system. A person must be sufficiently anchored in the system semantically. Immigrant children are faced with the demand that they also understand a second social system, which usually includes many sub-systems. There is some evidence that children can expand their cognitive performance greatly if given optimum opportunities, but otherwise the risk is obvious that the linguistic development becomes retarded and deficient.

The development of language is not only a question of learning from others. Rather, it is a creative process where the child from the very beginning is analyzing and checking words and sentences, playing with them, testing them on others, joking and inventing. This is a very important process if the language is to become a natural instrument for the production of thoughts. A person who has not been allowed to learn her/his mother tongue in this creative way will probably never feel really at ease when talking because the language will not have become part of her/his personality. The first years of life are most crucial with respect to linguistic learning. This is the time when the individual learns to know who she/he is, and what the world is like. This knowledge will remain all through life. We can fathom the bewilderment of an interrupted development and the hard work it demands if one language is brutally changed for another. Naturally, children can learn more than one language at a time or change over from one to another, but it takes much consideration and skill from the adults if it is to become a constructive process.

Learning the language of a new country is by no means an easy task because there is usually not one language but many. In every country, there are social groups, professions, age groups, and groups who develop their own terminology based on particular interests. The sexes use different phrases, according to recent research. There are different vernaculars within the same country, often with noticeable differences in words as well as in pronunciation. The language that is spoken by teachers and public speakers on radio and television is often very different from that used by the man in the street. There may be very great differences between the language that is spoken in the children's homes and the variety of idioms that they are expected to understand.

The semantic value of the words will also differ between the sub-groups, and the individual is supposed to know this. For example, one must know when it is proper to use polite phrases and when one may be less formal. A foreigner is usually allowed a little leeway, but there are rather narrow limits, especially among children and youth. It is very painful to trespass or to make a fool of oneself. Each culture stimulates the development of certain abilities and interests and inhibits others, and the languages reflect this. Many immigrants will experience that their previous knowledge is vastly insufficient, and that abilities that were cherished in the country of origin may not be appreciated. Because Swedish is taught by Swedes, there is generally no one to help immigrants to fill the gaps and to understand the differences. Although teachers may certainly do their best, they usually are knowledgeable only of their own culture, and there is plenty of mutual misconception between a teacher and the immigrant pupil.

Bilingualism is a pre-requisite for biculturalism, and hence linguistic deficiency is an obstacle on the road towards this state. But there are other problems connected to the upbringing of children in another country, problems that are connected to language but will here be discussed separately.

Many problems are due to the transition from one religion to another, or from cultures where religion plays an important role to another where it does not. A strict religion is one trait of an authoritarian pattern. When families leave the controlled and perhaps uncomfortably narrow atmosphere in their own country, they may feel relief but also anxiety. Their children may move away from their parents' beliefs without really acquiring others. If the children learn the new language more quickly than their parents, they may develop a feeling of superiority and disdain. This is felt as loss of prestige by the parents.

The identity development, which normally proceeds with parents and other members of the child's own group as models, will often be confused. The children feel more familiar with life in the new country and may well reject patterns of their parents' life. If the family comes from a country where corporal punishment is part of the pattern for upbringing, this may lead to serious consequences in Sweden, for example, where corporal punishment is forbidden by the law. Immigrant children often must adjust to an existence where they feel badly treated in comparison to Swedish children. They grow up in a country where the concept of freedom indeed is strongly manifested as regards individual rights to decide on one's own future. Such decisions are made not only on matters such as sexual debut, drinking habits, clothing and make-up, but also on marital status, studies, employment, political views, and so on. Confusion is a common state of mind for many immigrant children and their parents.

There will be clashes and conflicts in school. A Puerto-Rican teacher working in the United States tells about problems which certainly are similar to problems encountered in Sweden. A common topic for quarrel was time. Time, according to the Hispanic view, has no intrinsic value other than its requirements for human activity. You live your life as it comes, without planning ahead and without rushing from one activity to another. In the United States, as indeed Sweden, time value is diametrically opposite. Time is the master, and we are its slaves. We are expected to be spot on time, and anxious to know what to do weeks or months ahead. (Sueiro-Ross 1974.)

The Puerto-Rican children who were brought up to the Hispanic concept of time continuously found themselves in trouble when they were expected to react in the American way. Their teachers found them unbearably unable to comply with "normal" demands on punctuality. The teachers found the pupils recalcitrant or careless, and tried in vain to transform them into the time-stressed American pattern. The pupils who were culturally unequipped for this behaviour experienced the endless reprimands as evidence of their own worthlessness and inadequacy. The situation made life hopeless for both parties because both expected impossible reactions from each other.

Due to ignorance about each other's "self-evident facts", the teacher and the pupil continue to make life difficult for each other. Similar situations are common in every class where children from different cultures are expected to adjust to the host country's pattern of behaviour. In some cases, there are children from many different countries, and the poor teacher then will have to understand widely differing concepts. A less obvious, but nonetheless important, clash between cultures is that between Finnish and Swedish patterns of upbringing. The Finnish upbringing, however adequate it may be in the homeland, seems to engender among children in Sweden the fear of losing face. This frequently leads to passivity or extreme silence, and sometimes to mutism even among the pre-school ages. The situation has improved since education in Finnish was introduced, but a broad discussion among Finns is needed. If their ways of upbringing are causing their children problems, they ought to consider what changes might be necessary.

A very common problem among immigrant families is that of a child who learns her/his mother tongue up to the age of six or seven (depending on the compulsory school start) and who later is forced to change over more or less completely to the language of the majority society. If this child does not get aid with the further development of the first language, she/he may never be able to express her/himself in intellectual terms in the mother tongue, and will perhaps learn very little about the expressions of emotion and decision in the new language.

Genuine bilingualism should give the individual a good insight into more than one way of thinking, thereby broadening her/his views. A person who has learned only one way of thinking may easily become narrow-minded, unable to realize that there are different approaches to reasoning. This is due to the fact that languages are not neutral but laden with allusions, valuations and mutual know-how. Learning a new language and another culture is equal to learning new sets of truths. An adult may learn logically, comparing new views to old ones and hence keep her/his poise. A child, on the other hand, may be muddled and confused, unable to understand why rules differ and when to apply one behaviour or another.

An important factor to consider is that children are prone to learn by imitation. They may very quickly pick up enough to give an impression of being much more knowledgeable then they actually are. Many teachers in pre-school and the lower grades of compulsory school are led to think that linguistic ability is equal to the rather shallow understanding that is needed in peer group situations and its very limited number of requirements. They fail to observe that the children have not internalized all common associations of the words, that many words are understood only as parts of a context where complete understanding may be superfluous, or where the child may manage by pretending to understand. These gaps will widen unless teaching is truly skillful. Low understanding will lead to low motivation because incentives will be few and lessons dull.

Those who do not manage langage well enough will not learn well because language is both the tool of learning as well as the structure of the topics. A great many basic concepts are needed for coping with mathematics, for example, and if these are missing or confused, the pupil will learn instead that she/he is a bad learner. Gradually, when the school demands get heavier, the pupil will add to her/his feeling of being inadequate, of being one who cannot understand while others can.

Teachers must learn to understand that concepts need to be taught and to know how to remedy shattered egos. This is not an easy job, especially if the class is big and there are many other pupils who also need special tuition. There is a need for teachers and assistants who know the child's language so that some classes for Finnish pupils, for example, may be taught in Finnish, while other classes can have immigrant pupils mixed with Swedes. In Sweden, the number of home-language teachers is rapidly increasing, and attempts are being made to bring about a good team work in the schools. Much still remains to do, but there are many hopeful signs too.

Such team work is greatly needed from the very beginning, during pre-school age and onwards, if the immigrant children are to develop normally with respect to linguistic, emotional, and social growth. Many research workers have found a correspondence between problems of an emotional nature and linguistic inadequacy, the most common ones being extreme shyness, silence and submissiveness. There are also signs of the linguistic inadequacy getting worse instead of better when the children grow older. This includes deterioration in both the first language as well as the new language.

NOTE

* The ideas contained in this article were developed in the 'Dossiers for the Intercultural Training of Teachers. Sweden: the social/cultural situation of migrants and their families'.

(DECS/EGT (79) 122), published in 1980 by the Council for Cultural Cooperation of the Council of Europe.

REFERENCE

Sueiro-Ross
 1974 Cultural characteristics in bilingual learners. System 2, No. 2.

MARY ASHWORTH

THE CULTURAL ADJUSTMENT OF IMMIGRANT CHILDREN IN ENGLISH CANADA

IMMIGRATION TO CANADA

In the years prior to 1914 immigrants poured into this vastly underpopulated country of Canada. Western Europeans moved into the rapidly growing industrial cities of Ontario; Eastern Europeans broke open the prairie lands; and Japanese, Chinese and Indians took up fishing, mining, farming and lumbering in Canada's western province of British Columbia. Numbers dropped during the first World War but increased during the 1920's to fall once more during the depression days of the thirties. There was a difference, however, in the source countries as immigrants from Japan, China and India were almost totally excluded. With the end of hostilities following World War II, immigration picked up again, remaining fairly steady throughout the 1950's, dropping in the early 1960's and rising to its peak in the mid-1970's.

Post-war immigrants to Canada have consisted of three streams. The first stream comprised refugees: they came from war-torn Europe, from the revolutions in Hungary and Czechoslovakia, from Idi Amin's Uganda, from Chile and more recently from Viet Nam. A second stream consisted of independent immigrants and their families seeking a better life in a country which seemed to offer a measure of political, economic and personal freedom and prosperity. The last stream has borne the families of those who were already here and reunited them.

Since 1967 there has been another significant change in the major source countries, for in that year the Canadian government changed the immigration regulations so that they would apply equally to people of all races and nationalities. Discrimination against people from Asia, the West Indies and third-world countries was at an end with the introduction of a universal point system as the basis for acceptance. By the early 1970's immigration from India was twelve times what it had been only a few years before, and from Hong Kong, Taiwan and China it was fourteen times greater. Immigrants from English-speaking countries such as the United Kingdom and the U.S.A consequently represented a smaller proportion of the total immigration figure than in years gone by. By 1979 (the last year for which detailed statistics are available) close to three-quarters of the 112,096 men, women and children who immigrated to Canada came from non-English-speaking countries, and approximately one-third of these were children aged 0—19 years of age and therefore likely, at some time, to be enrolling in a school, college or university.

IMMIGRANT CHILDREN IN CANADIAN SCHOOLS

The first special classes for ESL (English as a Second Language) children were set up early in this century. Teachers and parents objected to the then current practice of placing older immigrant children in with six and seven year olds on the basis that if they spoke no English they must begin their schooling in grade one. But the education of immigrant children had neither priority nor prestige and was based on a policy of assimilation; and that was the way it remained until after World War II when a combination of increased immigration and a greater sensitivity towards immigrants engendered by the observed suffering of millions during the holocaust of the thirties and forties forced educators and governments to pay attention to the special needs of immigrant children.

The government of Ontario was the leader in the field. First, in the mid-1960's, it set up a program to train teachers to teach English as a second language to adults and children. Slowly, teacher-training institutions across Canada followed suit. Then it produced a two-volume ESL course for adults entitled *An Introduction to Canadian English* which, because there was no equivalent text for teachers of children, became the basic text for ESL classes in many public schools. Gradually, here and there large school districts appointed consultants to advise specialist ESL teachers and regular classroom teachers on how best to educate their New Canadian children, as they were then known.

In 1973, I conducted a survey to find out what the English-speaking provinces which received the bulk of the immigrants (British Columbia, Alberta, Saskatchewan, Manitoba and Ontario) were doing to facilitate the integration of non-English-speaking children into their various school systems. I found an anomaly. In a questionnaire, I asked ESL teachers what they thought was the major problem facing their ESL students. They indicated by a ratio of two to one that the major problem was not learning English but was, as one teacher put it, that of "coming to terms with the conflicting aspects of two cultures."[1] Another wrote, "They are caught between their parents' way of life and their new country's way. This often causes severe emotional and cultural problems."[2] But when I examined the goals of programs in which these children were enrolled, it was evident that the emphasis lay heavily on language learning with very little attention paid to cultural adjustment.

DEVIANT BEHAVIOUR PATTERNS

It was apparent to many teachers, then and now, that children who have difficulty adjusting to the Canadian school system or to life in Canada exhibit a variety of deviant behaviour patterns. Some children become extremely aggressive, creating many problems for themselves and for their teachers who try to curb their aggression. Others withdraw from the situation entirely, like one little boy who sat under his teacher's desk every day for three months before he finally agreed to take part in the normal classroom activities. Some children become listless, apathetic and tearful and are usually found on their own away from their classmates. Some find the struggle to achieve at a level near their potential is simply beyond them, and they give up and eventually drop out of school. Seeking a companionship not found in school, some join neighbourhood gangs and use the energy generated by their frustration in anti-social activities. In a deep desire to be accepted as Canadian, some children refuse to speak their home language and are ashamed of their parents when they speak their own tongue in public. This rejection by the child of the first language and culture can spell the beginning of a serious identity crisis. Some children go to the extreme of running away from home or attempting to commit suicide.

Children come to Canada from all over the world bringing with them widely different educational and cultural backgrounds. While children from any country may exhibit deviant behaviour patterns, those who settle down and do fairly well in school tend to be those who have come from an urban rather than a rural setting, who belong to the middle or professional class, and who come from very supportive homes where the parents are interested in having their children learn English and adopt Canadian customs. For those children who fail to adjust well to their new Canadian homeland, the causes of their deviant behaviour may lie in their inability to cope with their initial uprooting, or in what they have experienced in their homes, schools, or local communities since arriving in Canada.

1. *Uprooting*

Children can be deeply disturbed by the sudden loss of beloved relatives and friends; they may long for the familiar sights, sounds and smells of the past. Children do not always understand or accept the reasons given to them to justify moving to a new and strange land and may resent the decision made for them by their parents.

2. *The Home*

What goes on in the home deeply affects children. If the parents have difficulties adapting to a new life style, if they are worried, frustrated or unhappy, the children will sense this and become anxious too. If the family has not only moved from one country to another but has also moved from a rural to an urban setting, or, if owing to the high cost of living in Canada, the mother has, for the first time in her life, to seek employment outside the home, the sudden changes in familiar patterns and routines may further increase the tensions within the family. If the father switches jobs a number of times, or if the family frequently changes its place of residence, children may become quite unsettled. Children are also affected indirectly by the level of education and vocational training achieved by their parents prior to immigration to Canada and by their ability to speak English, as both factors will have a bearing on the kinds of jobs they can obtain and their ability to seek help when they need it. And then there is always the question: how much will the parents accept of the host country? Do they think that becoming a Canadian citizen is a worthwhile goal? Do they want their children to speak and act like Canadians? Are they prepared to see their children accept a value system different from their own? As one teacher put it, "They (the children) are caught between two cultures and torn between loyalty to the family and the need and desire to be integrated into the Canadian scene."[3]

3. *The School*

Children from abroad who enter a large concrete and glass urban Canadian school after attending a rural village school may be overwhelmed by its size as well as by the complexity of its program and general organization. Most children who come from non-English-speaking countries will have to learn the language of instruction; some will have to adjust to different teaching styles and different modes of learning. The level of some children's previous education may not be adequate for them to join a class of students of their own age thus creating a social problem. Because Canada is not without its bigots, some children may be hurt by discriminatory comments or acts by their classmates and their teachers. All these factors can build mounting tension in sensitive children.

The amount of parental support that children receive is therefore very important — the more the better. Unfortunately, a clash in values can occur between what schools say to children and demand of them and what parents will accept. There is also the matter of discipline. It is interesting to note that most teachers comment on how well immigrant children behave and how they wish all their students behaved as well, but some immigrant children interpret the relative freedom they find in Canadian classrooms as license to do whatever they please — with unhappy results.

A child who is the only one in the school who speaks a particular language or who belongs to a particular culture can experience a desperate state of isolation. On the other hand, children enrolled in schools containing a high percentage of students speaking the same language may have difficulty integrating with Canadian-born peers because divisions form along ethnic lines, and thus there is little opportunity for them to begin the process of stepping into the new society and making friends, and the period of alienation from those with whom they must eventually work and play is extended.

4. *The Community*

Both the children and their families can be hurt by the community around them if it is a cold, hostile community which fails to make the newcomers welcome and which offers them blank stares and derogatory comments instead of outstretched hands. There is no one more sensitive to the overt and covert intimations of rejection than a child.

Since 1973, the year of my survey, school districts and the provincial and federal governments have initiated various programs and actions which directly or indirectly have affected the cultural adjustment of immigrant children.

Unfortunately, it is not possible to offer any statistics to prove which of them has had the most beneficial effect on children because such statistics simply do not exist. However it is the "gut" feeling of a number of people working with immigrant children that many of the programs outlined below have the potential to cut down on the incidence of cultural maladjustment.

RECENT PROGRAMS AND ACTIONS

Because education is controlled by the provinces, program development in schools does not take place evenly across Canada. One province may be initiating a program that another province has just discarded. Wealthy provinces can provide seed money for pilot projects in schools and communities that poorer provinces must deny. Priorities are not the same across provinces. The position of the federal government in education remains somewhat of an anomaly. Under the British North America Act, the federal government is given no jurisdiction in education; however, it does fund many educational programs for adults and has given grants to the provinces to assist them in establishing programs for the teaching of French in English-medium schools. It has not supported the teaching of English to immigrant children, but it has supported a number of programs which have indirectly benefited these children.

It must be clearly understood, therefore, that the programs and actions described below are not ongoing in every part of Canada that has a sizable immigrant population, neither is their funding such that they will necessarily be ongoing a year from now. They do represent ways in which different school districts, municipalities, and provinces have tried to assist in the settlement, education and English language training of immigrant children and their families. These developments will be described under the same four headings used previously to outline the experiences that children live through after arriving in Canada.

1. *Uprooting*

It is beyond the power of the school to affect what happens to children before they arrive in Canada. However, the hiring of bilingual counsellors in schools and the availability of bilingual counselling services in public and private agencies in the community have made it easier for children and their families needing help to get it. School psychological services are also much more aware of the trauma that uprooting can bring and are also using bilingual psychologists and psychiatrists to work with difficult cases.

2. *The Home*

The need for the early orientation of the family to their new surroundings has been recognized and some programs established. Counselling and information services in the immigrant's own language are more readily available. The plight of the immigrant mother has received more attention. Special classes for mothers and their young children have been set up in some elementary schools, and classes are offered to help prepare women for the world of work. For those who cannot, for whatever reason, leave their homes, some cities offer in-house tutorial services. It is, of course, vital that the mental health and general welfare of the immigrant mother receive a high priority, as she can have a great influence on the way in which her children adjust to their new surroundings.

3. *The School*

There has been an improvement in the quality of pre-service training for ESL teachers over the past few years and an increase in its availability. Regular classroom teachers are more likely now to receive some insights into second language learning. While it is not mandatory for student-teachers to take specific courses dealing with multiculturalism in education, information along these lines is contained in other courses such as those dealing with educational psychology and sociology and the history of education. There has been a proliferation of in-service courses for practising teachers covering the backgrounds of the major ethnic groups found in schools and suggesting ways in which immigrant children can be helped to learn English and to adjust to the new culture.

ESL children are now less likely to be segregated in special classes located on the periphery of the school grounds and more likely to be integrated with their Canadian peers for at least part of the day in curricular and extra-curricular activities.

Some schools have made conscious efforts to hire bilingual teachers, particular counsellors; others have found funds to hire bilingual teacher aides and bilingual home-school workers. Children in these schools now have an adult they can talk to who understands their background and the trauma they are undergoing. Teachers, on the other hand, have someone they can refer to for information and advice on problems they have not previously encountered in their teaching careers.

There has been steadily growing awareness of the amount of racial and sexist stereotyping subtly displayed in textbooks, and strong efforts have been made to eradicate this. Teachers are more sensitive to the insidious racial prejudice still found in some schools, that is, unwarranted comments in the staffroom, name-calling on the playground and sometimes physical violence. Various teacher-groups are working to reduce the level of racism in schools, but so long as there is racism in local communities there will be a degree of racism in schools. As a more positive step, teachers of various subjects are being shown how they can incorporate a recognition of the multicultural nature of Canada in their lessons, and schools are encouraged to show an appreciation of the ethnic groups represented in the schools by suitably marking ethnic holidays and festivities. The province of Ontario has launched a Heritage Language Program which allows schools to play a role in the maintenance of the children's home language. Measures which strengthen children's sense of identity and which enable them to add another language and another culture without losing what they bring to Canada should produce young adults able to work and play comfortably in two languages and two cultures.

4. *The Community*

Canada has its racists who, in times of high unemployment and inflation, try to lay the blame for the country's ills on the backs of the immigrants. Various levels of government have, from time to time, put on advertising campaigns or run educational programs to try to combat the poisoned words of the racists. The press has also become more responsible in the way in which it deals with immigration and racism in its columns. The federal government, a few years ago, established its own advisory group, the Canadian Consultative Council on Multiculturalism, and also contracted several writers to produce histories of the trials and successes of the many ethnic groups in Canada. In this way it is recognizing the valuable contribution of ethnic groups other than English or French to the growth and development of the nation.

Because children belong to a number of different communities, the family, the school, the neighbourhood, the church, the ethnic group and so on, the task of assisting them to make a healthy adjustment to Canada is not the responsibility of the school alone, but is one which also devolves onto the larger society. While recent developments are encouraging, an imperfect world remains imperfect and we have to be thankful that in spite of poor services or a lack of empathy, the resilience of children and the inner fortitude they bring with them from their homelands give many of them the strength to overcome the difficulties facing them and to make a successful adjustment.

NOTES

[1] N. M. Ashworth, *Immigrant Children and Canadian Schools*, Toronto: McClelland and Stewart, 1975, p. 125.
[2] Ibid.
[3] Ibid.

BEVERLY NANN, B.A., B.S.W.

SETTLEMENT PROGRAMS FOR IMMIGRANT WOMEN AND FAMILIES

Among new immigrant families settling in North America today, wives and mothers comprise a group with problems and needs which differ significantly from those of other members of a migrant population. Many of these women come from background cultures where the adult female role is highly circumscribed when compared with the relative freedom enjoyed by their counterparts in North American society. Despite the greater opportunities for personal development existing in their new environment, immigrant women are often condemned to a restricted life style that is enclosed in a psycho-cultural structure mirroring the society which they have left behind. This life style is particularly prevalent when an immigrant family settles in an ethnic community exhibiting institutional completeness (Breton, 1964). Able to fulfill their psychosocial needs within a community having similarities to the one from which they have left, people may remain within it, participating very little with the majority culture, clinging to traditional values or practices, and perhaps never learning the language of their adopted country. Immigrant men have greater opportunities to escape such a life style because pressures to earn a living usually force the adult male into greater contact with the larger society. However, many immigrant women, and particularly mothers with young children, find themselves with no equivalent opportunities for a different way of life.

An oft expressed sentiment of immigrant parents is that they have come to North America seeking a better future for their children, and they come prepared to sacrifice their own happiness for the sake of their children's future. My question is — why must these parents sacrifice their own lives for their children; are these immigrant parents not also entitled to a rich, full life for themselves? In my view, once an immigrant has gained entry into North America, then we, as hosts, have a responsibility to extend a helping hand to assist in easing and facilitating the newcomer to become a full participant in our society.

This paper will examine two outreach projects in the city of Vancouver that respond to the settlement needs of immigrant families. The first, known as the Immigrant Resources Project, developed as a response to the special settlement problems of young immigrant mothers and their preschool-aged children. The second program is known as the Multicultural Home-School Liaison Project which addresses itself to the larger group of immigrant families with school-aged children who today comprise some 43% of the total Vancouver student population (24,727 of a total student population of 57,505). The development of these projects were guided by three basic concepts:

(1) All immigrants who come to Canada share some common settlement experiences;

(2) A transitional service based on a bilingual and bicultural approach (i.e., Anglo-Canadian and the immigrant's own language and culture) can ease the settlement process and facilitate and accelerate the integration of immigrants into Canadian life;

(3) A school-based service is an effective and efficient way of reaching families with children in this age group.

COMMON SETTLEMENT EXPERIENCES

In my work with immigrant populations in Vancouver over the past five years, I have noted that various groups, regardless of their cultural background, exhibit many common characteristics. For the most part, family interests seem to take precedence over the interests of any individual member; parenting practices tend to be authoritarian and conservative; and a strong extended-family system functions as a social support network. As they settle into Canadian society, similar stresses and strains are experienced. Generally speaking, the process of settlement would seem to include the following elements:

An Uprooting Period: Immigrants experience both a psychological as well as a physical move. For many, it means the breaking of deep, meaningful ties which may go back for several hundreds of years into history. I think of my grandfather leaving his ancestral home for Canada. He came from a Chinese village which was settled over 1100 years ago, and family records show him as the 26th generation descended from the original founders of the village. Imagine leaving this familiar world for the unknown. It is difficult enough for Canadians to move from one part of Canada to another — how much more difficult it must be for an immigrant to move from one culture to another.

The Rural-Urban Adjustment: Immigrants who come from a rural background such as the villages of Greece or the Punjab are accustomed to a relatively simple society where everyone has a place and no one feels a stranger. Becoming immersed into a complex, impersonal, urban society can be confusing, overwhelming, and disorienting. It is little wonder that many are drawn into their own ethnic communities for comfort and support.

Culture Shock: In the case of most immigrant groups, there is little or no preparation for the challenge to their traditional values and way of life as they encounter Canadian society. Our emphasis on individualism, the rights of women and children, the liberal attitudes toward parenting, education, courtship and marriage, and the extensive network of community social services replacing the extended family support system — all of these things are alien and threatening to many immigrants.

Loss of Familiar Social Supports: Many immigrants come from societies where one's daily life was closely shared among family members and friends. Such persons were easily accessible and available. Contrast this to the case of an economically well-established East Indian family who is presently considering a move back to India after nine years in Canada because the parents miss the rich, meaningful social life they enjoyed in the old country. They have found Canadian friendships to be shallow and non-committed, prompting the comment, "Of what use is our big, beautiful home here when no one comes to visit?" With this void comes a feeling of isolation and loneliness.

Change of Economic and Social Status: Many immigrants have professional training which is not recognized in Canada. Lack of language fluency, an absence of Canadian work experience and the current high level of unemployment in the country are factors which lead to the under-employment of immigrant workers. Economic necessity, along with opportunities for employment for women are factors which encourage immigrant mothers to enter the work force, bringing about a major change in the adult female role which, in turn, affects relationships among other members of the family.

Discrimination and Intolerance: Immigrant groups, particularly those who may be described as visible minorities, are often the target of discrimination, misunderstanding, and intolerance. These negative aspects of Canadian society are reinforced by the currently depressed economic conditions where the new immigrant, typically, becomes an easy scapegoat.

In addition to the kinds of experiences mentioned thus far which all immigrants share to a greater or less degree, families with young children in the home are likely to confront further types of difficulties. These include:

Parenting Dilemmas: Many immigrant parents are caught between the strict and authoritarian discipline of their native culture and the more democratic and consultative approach to child rearing in North America. The children of immigrant families may be under pressure to maintain their ethnic values and culture which are often in conflict with value systems encountered outside of the home. When grandparents are in the home, they may find their traditional authority challenged, and indeed, the older generation often find themselves totally dependent upon their children for the very first time. Some grandparents are brought over to Canada to help care for young ones in the home. These persons usually have little motivation to change their ways and are heavily dependent upon their immediate families to meet all of their needs. Parents then are caught between trying to satisfy grandparents and responding to the needs of their children. Children may come to have power over their non-English speaking parents. As children are apt to be quicker in learning the language of a new society, they may control the communication from school, for example, and from the surrounding English-speaking community.

Generation Communication Gap: As immigrant children enter Canadian schools, the ethnic language may begin to recede in importance to them. If, at the same time, adults in the home fail to learn English, effective communication between family members becomes increasingly difficult. It is frustrating and at times impossible to communicate with any great sensitivity or diplomacy.

Adapting to a New Educational System: Many immigrant families, conditioned to a culture which separates the school from the home, encounter great difficulty with a Canadian school system which promotes parental involvement and fosters the social as well as the academic development of the student. When a note comes home from the school, the first reaction is that something is wrong and their child is in some kind of trouble. In many cases, the opportunity for children to have a better education was a factor in the family's migration, and this can lead to immense pressures upon immigrant children to do well in school.

Adolescent Identity Crises: Young members from immigrant homes often feel trapped between two cultures, wondering which values to accept or reject. A feeling of distance develops as they become better educated than their parents. Some become ashamed of their heritage and even of their own family, but this may only exacerbate their search for a comfortable self-identity.

BRIDGING SERVICES FOR FAMILIES IN TRANSITION

Many immigrants do successfully resettle with very little help from the rest of us. Nevertheless, it has been my experience that they all deeply appreciate a friendly helping hand. Then, there are those who do not have the resources or experience to deal effectively with the kinds of problems and dilemmas mentioned earlier in this paper. For them, there is the need for help to ease and encourage their integration into Canadian life.

We value the contributions made by immigrants to our economy but generally overlook the greater contribution they can make to all spheres of Canadian society when they feel a part of the mainstream. Successful integration and settlement of newcomers is a two-way process, requiring active interaction of both established Canadians and newcomers. Both need to be aware, sensitive, and tolerant of cultural differences and be prepared for adjustments and compromises where conflicting values are involved.

My experience suggests that service programs for immigrant families and children are most effective when they are established on what might be termed a bicultural and bilingual model. In other words, the staff and the volunteers who service these programs should include members who come from the same cultural backgrounds as the immigrant users of service. This not only enhances the quick development of an initial trust necessary for effective intervention but also makes it more likely that the program personnel will understand the strengths of their clients' background, traditions, cultural aspirations, concerns and conflicts. Established immigrants who have made a good adaptation have proved to be invaluable resources. They serve as a role model for other immigrants, and as a link to connect clients to program services, local schools, and other community resources.

As the school system extends into almost all sections of the community, a school-based program is in a unique position to reach out to assess, monitor, and respond to the special needs of immigrant families and children. Our experience in Vancouver has confirmed the fact that immigrants have a high regard for schools. Immigrants will readily accept services offered through the school while shying away from help offered by other governmental or non-governmental agencies. Some immigrants may even refuse to approach their own ethnic organizations for help because of a loss of face within their own ethnic community. Moreover, there are, during the course of a normal school year access points into an immigrant family to discuss, for example, a child's academic progress, his or her health concerns, or a parent's participation in a special school event. Finally, the compulsory period of school attendance in our society makes it possible to have a continuity of contact with immigrant families while their children are enrolled in the educational system.

TWO EXAMPLES OF BILINGUAL, BICULTURAL SCHOOL-BASED PROGRAMS

(A) *The Immigrant Resources Project*

This program began as a response to the settlement needs of Chinese immigrant women living in Vancouver and to concerns expressed by school officials over the special problems of their children. Started in 1975 with the support of government, community, and volunteer groups, this program has since extended to serve seven different immigrant populations, the largest being Chinese, East Indian, Italian and Greek. A variety of activities is provided by paid staff and volunteers designed particularly for non-English speaking mothers who are known to be isolated from the larger Canadian society. The program includes a head start educational component for preschool immigrant children in order to place them on an equal footing with their Canadian peers by the time they begin their formal schooling. Some basic English language training for the mothers is also an integral part of the program, along with activities which help to integrate the mothers and children into our general Canadian society.

The programmed activities are primarily based on group experiences where immigrant mothers and their young children can have the support and comfort of sharing with other members of their own ethnic group. The various groups come together at least twice a week over an eight-months period, which corresponds approximately to the regular school year. This educational orientation, among other things, is important to the fathers of many immigrant families who are ready to allow their wives and youngsters to participate in learning activities, whereas a program identified as a social service may meet with resistance.

Underlying this program are the following assumptions:

(1) a bilingual, bicultural approach is essential for non-English speaking immigrants if communication is to be effective and meaningful; this allows the immigrant to participate in activities to the extent to which she is capable and desires to do so;

(2) achieving some fluency in English is essential if the immigrant is going to be able to step beyond her own ethnic community in any meaningful way;

(3) initially, non-English speaking immigrants need a social support group, comprising people of their own ethnic background (to replace the social support network severed in emigrating) to meet their social and mutual aid needs (something familiar and comfortable in a strange new world);

(4) given a supportive, encouraging environment, immigrants can develop the confidence to cope with the larger community and become more actively involved, contributing members of Canadian society;

(5) immigrants need to be introduced and oriented to Canadian life and resources to facilitate their integration into Canadian society;

(6) people learn best through "first-hand" experiences in matters that are immediate to them in their daily lives;

(7) the children of immigrant families also need to be prepared for life in Canada;

(8) it is important to protect the integrity of the family by involving all of its members, especially the husbands whenever possible; the orientation experience will have greater impact if the family is involved and supportive.

Elements of the Program

The Immigrant Resources Project comprises a variety of activities. These include:

(a) Social, cultural, community orientation and citizenship activities;

(b) Bilingual "headstart" English instruction for the adult;

(c) Headstart preschool experiences for the younger children, with child care services provided for the very young;

(d) Social support services;

(e) School orientation activities;

(f) Cultural exchanges with representatives of different ethnic groups.

(a) *Social, Cultural, Community Orientation and Citizenship Activities*: This component of the program provides an introduction to key community services available in Canada, and exposes immigrants to Canadian cultural traditions such as the celebration of Thanksgiving, Christmas, and Easter. In responding to the practical needs of clients, there are demonstrations and discussion on such things as the Canadian standards of personal hygiene, and the North American practice of packing school lunches for students.

(b) *Bilingual "Headstart" English Instruction*: This component provides a non-threatening and supportive approach to English instruction for adults with emphasis on engendering the necessary confidence for successful language learning. Most of the clients will be at a very beginning level and the first step is to provide them with what might be called "survival English" so that they may cope with everyday living. A bilingual approach is used to ease the transition to English. Gradually, the translation service is withdrawn so that by the end of the year, an English immersion approach is used in preparation for "graduation" into a formal unilingual English class which is available at various sources in the community.

(c) *Headstart Pre-School Experience for 3 and 4 Year Olds*: This activity serves to facilitate the eventual involvement of immigrant children in kindergarten and school life. Play activities are used which will stimulate the use of English language, and a sound preschool experience is provided based on the Cooperative Preschool Model with its strong parent education focus, but adapted to the special needs of immigrant families. Bilingual services are available as required to comfort the children. Volunteers who themselves have English-speaking preschoolers are recruited to help in this program. The children of the volunteers encourage the use of English among the immigrant youngsters, and provide a role model for immigrant preschoolers who are often reluctant to attempt strange new activities. A vital aspect of this program is the provision of child care services for the very young. This makes it possible for all mothers to participate, and also meets the need of immigrant parents who traditionally take their children everywhere with them.

(d) *Social Support Services*: These include individual, family and group counselling services, and the use of an ethnic group social support network. Short-term individual counselling and referral services are provided for personal adjustment problems. Group counselling is used to deal with common problems and concerns among several families where the sharing of experiences, concerns, and possible solutions can be reassuring and supportive, and help counter feelings of alienation and discouragement. The group support network attempts to replace the social and family relationships severed in migration, by creating a caring, supportive community which will provide ongoing mutual aid activities and enduring friendships among its members.

(e) *School Orientation Activities*: For immigrant families with children in the home, the successful adaptation to Canadian schools is a vital part of their overall settlement in this country. As the Immigrant Resources Project is itself a school-based program, many opportunities arise to link immigrant families to their local school system. The concept here is to encourage the families to develop a full and active participation in the educational life of their children.

(f) *Cultural Exchanges*: Non-English speaking immigrants in Canada generally have limited opportunities for exposure to other cultural groups who make up our Canadian mosaic. Cultural exchanges are organized between different cultural groups within the Project to promote understanding and tolerance of other cultures, which is an essential part of learning to live in a multicultural Canada. The regular exchanges between Canadian volunteers in the program and the immigrant clientele are also meaningful to both.

(B) *The Multicultural Home/School Liaison Project*

This Project developed out of the concern among several agencies in the community about the special needs of the 43% of students within the Vancouver school system who come from homes where English is a second language. The major focus of the Home/School Liaison service is to bridge the gap between the immigrant home and school, and between home and community. As in the Immigrant Resources Project, the programs here involve the use of bilingual and bicultural workers who are directly familiar with the ethnic cultures represented in the persons of the immigrant families served by this Project.

It is often the case that a Home/School worker first makes contact with a family through the request of a school official, such as a teacher or a psychologist, who is unable to help a student with a problem because of language or cultural barriers. As families find themselves helped this way with school problems, they subsequently take the initiative in turning to the Home/School workers with problems beyond the school.

The range of services provided by our Home/School workers may involve one or a combination of the following: orientation to school and community for students and parents; interpretation services, including translation of school materials; pre-kindergarten orientation services; short-term student or parent counselling; referral to community services; encouragment of parent involvement in the school and in community activities; adult education on topics such as English instruction, career development, and parenting; cultural enrichment; social adjustment and self-identification groups for students; multicultural exchanges and cultural sensitization of school personnel and the local community.

During the past two years, a total of 17 multicultural workers have been employed in this Project to serve immigrant families within the school system. The workers operate as a cultural resource, providing a vital communication link between school personnel, the immigrant families, and other contacts in the community.

In summary, as a self-proclaimed multicultural society, Canada's major institutions have been slow to respond to the multicultural fact and to the need to "multiculturalize" our service delivery systems. In both of the projects described in this paper, the workers and volunteers are filling some of the service gaps for families and children who come from a variety of cultural backgrounds. The combined experience of these programs points to the value of supportive, transitional services to help bridge immigrants to the Canadian mainstream, and these services have received the unanimous support of key organizations and groups within the ethnic communities themselves and of major systems in the larger society such as government, school, and non-governmental community agencies and groups.

By providing these educational, social support services, we not only strengthen the immigrant families and thereby our total society, we also help to minimize the disorientation that often comes with an uprooting experience and to prevent the development of serious mental health disorders. Coincidentally, we are raising the consciousness of the host community toward the needs and aspirations of immigrant groups. In the process, we not only benefit from their contributions to our economic well-being but our sociocultural fabric is also strengthened and enriched through the increased involvement of immigrants in all spheres of Canadian life.

REFERENCES

Ashworth, Mary N.
    1975 Immigrant Children in Canadian Schools. McClelland and Stewart, Toronto.

Breton, Raymond
    1964 Institutional completeness of ethnic communities and the personal relations of immigrants. American Journal of Sociology 70, September.

Nann, Beverly
    1978 Immigrant Resources Project Manual. Immigrant Services Society, Vancouver, September.

Vancouver School Board
    1979 The Multicultural Home/School Workers Project. Evaluation and Research Services, September.

BEN CHUD, M.S.W.

THE THRESHOLD MODEL: A CONCEPTUAL FRAMEWORK FOR UNDERSTANDING AND ASSISTING CHILDREN OF IMMIGRANTS

A great deal of interest in migration and immigration settlement exists throughout the world. Sociologists, psychologists, social workers, and psychiatrists have engaged in research and produced papers related to migration and immigration. Case histories have been collected. Statistical data have been gathered, and studies related to government policies and infrastructures dealing with immigrants proliferate.

What has not been so evident are efforts given to the creation of conceptual models which would be of assistance in helping professionals in their work with recently arrived immigrants. Yet without such models, the helping professional is left to deal with these immigrants as though they were native-born clients. Of course, the helping person takes into account cultural and language differences. But having done so, he then proceeds to employ such models and techniques which are familiar to him. Without doubt, much of what we know about human behavior and forms of intervention are universal. And to the extent that this is so, the helping professional may be well served by prevailing intervention approaches. On the other hand, there is the persistent and nagging thought that an additional conceptual framework would be of assistance. This paper is intended as a contribution in that direction.

Over and over again, and wherever we turn, we receive confirmation of the adaptability of human beings both old and young. Immigrants move from tropical and warm weather climates to countries with severe winters, and the vast majority of them are able to accommodate to varying degrees. The same is true in reverse. Likewise, these immigrants adapt to different cultures, agricultural and industrial modes, language, custom and economic standards of life. This is important to stress so that we can maintain a balanced view of immigrant populations. Indeed, the issues and problems confronting immigrants do not necessarily require professional intervention as, fortunately, large numbers of immigrants are able to cope with their new situations.

If the above is true of most adult immigrants, then it is even truer for children of immigrant parents for the adaptability quotient of children is even greater than that of adults. Experts who have studied the language acquisition of people have concluded that children acquire new languages more readily than do most adults. Moreover, children are still in the formative stage of socialization and are, therefore, more susceptible, amenable, and malleable to new ideas and behaviours than are adults.

Another characteristic of immigrant settlement is that whenever one looks at the phenomenon of mass migration, one finds that when the host country makes it possible for the immigrant group to freely choose its own geographic location,

R. C. Nann (ed.), Uprooting and Surviving, 95–99.
Copyright © *1982 by D. Reidel Publishing Company.*

then the immigrants tend to band together in certain areas of a city or town. This "free choice" is not always as free as one might suppose. Most frequently, the reasons for the creation of an immigrant section or community are definitely rooted in the economics of the situation. Thus, the density of immigrant groups in certain localities is dictated by the amount of money available for rent, etc. Then again, there are situations where the employment of the immigrant group is such as to determine where they live in terms of proximity to their work place. Thus, we have on the one hand the human potential for great adaptability and on the other a reduced need to adapt because immigrant groups frequently live in such compact masses that they can in considerable measure maintain and replicate their own cultures.

Of necessity, these preliminary remarks have been brief. Yet, they constitute the foundation to that which I call the Threshold Model. The dictionary describes a threshold as "the entrance or beginning point of something", or "the point at which a stimulus is just strong enough to be perceived or produce a response." Both of these definitions are useful in elaborating this model.

The home of the immigrant family usually vibrates with the culture of the country of origin. If the immigrant family lives in an area densely populated by members of the same immigrant group, then the street or streets will not differ greatly from the home of the individual family. Still, there comes a threshold point, that is, the point at which there is a "beginning of something new" or a "point at which the stimulus is just strong enough to be perceived or produce a response". In some cases then, the threshold may be crossed at the front door of the immigrant family and in others, it will be at the point at which the particular community is cheek by jowl with the citizens of the host country. But whether one is speaking of individual family home or a compact community, members will cross the threshold to varying degrees. The very young, the elderly, and the non-employed adult do so less frequently than do those who are at work. Children of school age confront the threshold phenomenon each and every day as they go to school. These children come face to face with the host culture to the greatest degree. The challenges they face are linguistic, academic, and social. There is also the challenge to their value system.

Just as the immigrants are called upon to cross backwards and forwards over the threshold, so do members of the host country. This occurs both formally and otherwise. A multitude of systems make themselves felt on the immigrants. The list is almost endless and for illustrative purposes only I make mention of but a few. These include: customs and immigration departments, reception agencies, the media, advertising, observed clothing differences, games, recreation places, social agencies, and so on. The legal system, including leases, contracts, insurance, taxes of all kinds, and deductions from wages, are not the least of these since they frequently call for a level of abstraction and novelty previously not encountered.

The notion of "threshold" is therefore one way of conceptualizing the intricacies of the interface between the immigrant and the host country. Because this paper is intended for a workshop given over to children of immigrants, I propose to develop the model as it applies to school age children.

In this connection, I conceive the idea of the threshold as falling into three categories. The first might be thought of as the relatively Unobstructed Threshold. In this situation, the child crosses from the home culture into the larger world with little difficulty. Both the school and the home are congenial and complementary one to other. Teachers, peers, counsellors and the entire school ambience are supportive to the child. There is a patient and understanding attitude towards language acquisition. A positive attitude is adopted towards the child's first language. There is a display of respect to various cultures. There is, above all, a willingness to be flexible and innovative on the part of the system. As the child crosses back over the threshold into the home, he or she is confronted with keen curiosity and interest by the people at home. The child in this situation is seen not only as a learner but also as a transmitter — a go-between — of the two cultures. Such an attitude is of service to the ego of the child since the child is given, and takes on, an important function in the family.

The second threshold category is perhaps best described as the Problematic Threshold. A variety of factors may contribute to such a state of affairs. By way of illustration, I suggest that the isolated immigrant child is a likely candidate. Being one of very few students in a school who are immigrants and perhaps the only one in a particular class makes the child vulnerable. No one to share with, and no one to play with, might be characteristic of such a situation. The extreme minority status of the child may lead to benevolent neglect on the part of the system. Meanwhile, back at home, all of this is not without consequence. One possible reaction on the part of the family is to close ranks, move into isolation and find solace in segregation and mutual support. While I have confined myself to a single illustration of the Problematic Threshold, I feel certain that those of you who have worked with children and families of immigrants can provide a great deal of additional rich material.

The final category is one I have labelled the Traumatic Threshold. Contributing to this state of affairs might be such elements as a rigid educational system, acts of racial discrimination which result in fear of going to school and returning back to the home, insulting graffiti, and labelling students as "slow learners" or children with learning problems when, in fact, the problems are elsewhere — overcrowded conditions at home, lack of understanding about extracurricular activities at school, which means that the child is, in the eyes of their parents, staying away from the home without good reason, expectations of the school on the part of the parents which are not being met, and the corrupting influences which, as the parents see it, are being manifested by their offspring. It is not, of course, necessary for all of these factors to be operative in order that the Traumatic Threshold situation should prevail. One, or a combination of several, could produce such results.

The Unobstructed, the Problematic and the Traumatic Thresholds all have implications for the human service practitioner. For the practitioner engaged in community development and policy planning, each of these categories represents a challenge. A congenial school system does not happen by and of itself. School authorities at the highest level are in need of guidance and preparation. Policies as to special courses, and resources for the teaching of a second language cannot be left to chance. Financial backup needs to be provided so that good intention moves to practical application. Teachers need to be sensitized to the needs and the culture of the immigrant child. Home-school liaison personnel is a vital necessity, and school counsellors have a vital role to play. Home-school organizations where immigrant parents can feel comfortable involve careful planning. Provision needs to be made for circulars, letters and other forms of publicity in the first language of the immigrant parents. Creating vital links in the ethnic community forms part of the work of such practitioners. Above all, what is required is the involvement of the parents of these children in planning and action.

Hopefully, the policies and preparation for immigrant children in a school district will be made in anticipation of the arrival of such children. More often than not such activity, if taken at all — and in a good many places no such preparation is even contemplated — occurs after the fact of immigrant arrival.

What is important to stress is that the onus of responsibility for the creation of a congenial threshold is upon the host country and not on the immigrants. Therein lies the hub and nub of the issue. For in countries where immigrants are viewed negatively because of economic considerations, racial prejudice (and the two are often linked), or because of cultural differences, the host is not likely to expend financial and/or human resources in order to ease the transitional stage of the immigrants. But even in countries where a more positive attitude prevails towards the newcomers, there may still be the position taken that the sooner these people are assimilated, the better for all concerned. This latter approach overlooks the deep-rootedness of culture. One has only to study countries where the bulk of the population is made up of immigrants — and my own country, Canada, is in this category — to find that important aspects of the country of origin still manifest themselves after five and even more generations are born in Canada. Thus, it is evident that cultural roots run deep. In some cases, they find expression in linguistic terms but, more frequently than not, they are to be perceived in celebration of holidays, maintenance of various cultural traditions, and adherence to organizations, church groups and the like.

For the mental health worker or counsellor, the Problematic and Traumatic Threshold concepts may in the first instance be useful because of its focus on environmental considerations. Individuals or family members are viewed as having difficulties with coping because of the stresses and challenges to their values, mores and traditions, as well as the demands of learning a new language, seeking employment, acquiring new ways of earning a livelihood, etc. In a word, the emphasis is on conditions of living rather than on personal pathology. In order that the worker might be effective around "conditions of life", he or she must acquire knowledge about both sides of the threshold. The worker must know the school, its administration, members of the staff, and resources in the school.

The worker must develop a good working relationship with the school. On the other side, unless the worker is of the same cultural background as the immigrant client, it would be foolhardy to suggest the possibility of gaining instant expertise. But what is called for is a heightened sensitivity on the part of the professional.

We have all encountered somewhere in the literature the idea that we need to respect our clients even if we do not like their behaviour. In the case of immigrants, this concept requires modification. I would suggest that heightened sensitivity means that we respect our clients and want to understand their behaviour.

The model calls upon the worker to engage in three fundamental tasks. These tasks apply equally on both sides of the threshold. The first is information giving. When there is a gap in information, misunderstanding results. Lack of information is frequently replaced by misinformation. This makes for difficulties in crossing the threshold. Secondly, the worker has the task of educating. Again, I am concerned with the educational tasks which address each side of the threshold. Education includes fact and data but goes beyond these to incorporate ways of thinking about issues. Education is concerned with the why and way to get there. Thirdly, the worker along with the clients in both systems need to undertake environmental manipulation. This may involve physical changes in areas such as housing; attitudinal changes by teachers, parents and students in the class; or administrative changes in the school's way of communicating with the parents.

No part of what I have written is to be taken as a denial of the fact that some immigrant children are indeed suffering from psychological and emotional problems. Such children and their families are, of course, in need of specialized treatment. But even in these cases, the threshold concept ought to be taken into account.

The Threshold Model is intended to highlight two systems and their interface as it applies to school age immigrant children, i.e., the individual family or immigrant community on the one hand, and the school of the other. It involves preventative, habilitative and treatment functions. The model is in my view sufficiently broad so that other segments of the immigrant population and the host country can be incorporated but this would take us outside of the scope of our present discussion.

GEORGE V. COELHO, Ph.D.

THE FOREIGN STUDENT'S SOJOURN AS A HIGH RISK SITUATION: THE "CULTURE-SHOCK" PHENOMENON RE-EXAMINED

When young people move to a new culture for a period of intensive education abroad, they are exposed to many complex changes in their environment to which they must readily adapt in order to function effectively. Foreign students, especially from old cultures in developing countries, may undergo a double uprooting process. The first uprootedness is when they are transplanted from their habitat to the new industrialized and technological environment, and the second is when, after several years of study abroad, they face relocation and re-entry into more or less traditional patterns of their home society. Worldwide rapid changes in an urbanizing planet (Coelho and Stein, 1977) tend to increase the kinds of uprooted populations around the world, of which foreign students are a high risk group (Alexander, 1976; WHO, 1977). This paper examines the major stressful elements of high risk situations involved in the transition of students to a foreign culture. It suggests a framework for identifying key factors in transition situations of study abroad. It examines the culture shock phenomenon in terms of major emotional issues of *loss* experienced in the stresses of uprootedness; and finally it discusses some practical applications for orientation and counselling programs that may be designed to facilitate coping strategies and social adaptation of foreign students.

A coping model of adaptive behavior has been used for examining stressful transitions in the life cycle (Coelho, Hamburg & Adams, 1974), such as the child's first school experience, the junior school transition, the transition from high school to college, graudate student stress, etc. Education abroad is a major developmental and psychosocial transition in a foreign student's life. Like other transitions, it represents a series of phases of high risk situations that produce emotional stress as well as opportunities for coping behavior.

The concept of coping is used to refer to psychosocial adaptation under unusually difficult circumstances (White, 1974). In transition situations, the individual is required to meet simultaneously many new tasks of adaptation in a coordinated way within a time frame. In order to be able to cope, the individual in a foreign environment must be able to do the following:

1. to gain adequate information — neither ignorance nor overload is useful;

2. to maintain satisfactory internal conditions, including effective regulation of physiological functions and of emotional distress;

3. to maintain autonomy, or a certain freedom of action — avoiding, on the one hand, the danger of "only one way", and on the other, the disaster of "no way out".

Studies of stressful transitions in the life cycle have shown that coping behavior usually serves the following functions: it helps to maintain a sense of personal worth and self-esteem, to maintain continuity of relationships with significant others, to maintain distress and tension within manageable limits.

The concept of *high risk* is derived from the field of public health promotion and is applied to characteristics of a group profile rather than to particular individuals (Lalonde, 1974). Thus, for example, males between 40 and 70 in the United States are particularly susceptible to death from coronaries, or as they are popularly known, "heart attacks". Within this population, the typical high risk profile would indicate an obese person who gets little or no exercise, eats excessive amounts of animal fats, drinks lots of coffee, works long hours in a high pressure job, etc. Such men are candidates for coronaries. Risk is a statistical term which is expressed in percentages or odds. Thus a man with a high risk group profile is more likely than a man with a low risk group profile to die from a heart attack.

The concept of risk cannot be used to make predictions about particular individuals. However, it helps to focus attention on population groups who are exposed to stressful situations at a vulnerable period in their career and development.

Reviewing the foreign student literature from this perspective it is possible to derive group profiles of high risk and low risk foreign student populations, to plot specific stressful situations associated with various phases of the sojourn abroad, and to link these situations to stages of the individual's development.

Several indices of risk have been suggested by Klineberg (1980) in his discussion of non-academic criteria for education abroad, e.g. language competence, advance knowledge of the culture, psychological preparation, coping abilities, etc.

A matrix of group profiles can be thus prepared which will locate not only vulnerability factors but also competence and coping factors for each phase of the sojourn of different student populations. The "culture shock" phenomenon and the "U-Curve hypothesis" have been well documented in the literature. However, they need to be examined in greater detail for the *meaning* of these experiences in the individual's psychosocial development.

The double U-Curve representing the changes in levels of satisfaction from the first phse of arrival in the new environment to the re-entry to the home environment, can be interpreted in terms of the double uprooting process. The trough of depression has been identified in the U-Curve hypothesis, but the nature and the effects of this trough have not been analyzed in terms of specific stressful situations that may be common or unique to specific student populations from developing countries. What are key dimensions of risk, such as duration, intensity, amplitude or depth? It is important to know whether the trough is short or prolonged. Is it shallow or deep? Did it appear suddenly or slowly? Is it steady or fluctuating? A prolonged, severe, steadily deepening trough of depression would characterize a high risk group profile in a given foreign student population.

The trough of depression in the U-Curve represents a risk situation, but its meaning and effect on a given individual will depend on several factors: his vulnerability in terms of the specific stress situations in his academic and cultural environment, the social support systems available and used, and his preparatory experiences of coping with new and unfamiliar situations in his own society.

For each phase of the sojourn, high risk situations can be identified, probable stressful events mapped out, and diverse coping strategies illustrated. For purposes of discussion, let us take an example of the *precursor* conditions and preparatory experiences that contribute to high risk situations in the sojourn of Indian students in the United States.

Indian students come to the United States prepared to use adaptive strategies which they have learned in a certain environment that is characteristically very different from the American academic and cultural milieu in which they have to survive and cope. The following family and culture patterns are typical of the socialization process of Indian students:

1. The young Indian grows up usually surrounded by a large household of older and younger members, relatives, and servants in which the parental figures and sometimes grandparents play a visible, important and pervasive role.

2. Children are early prepared to recognize their place in the family's hierarchical social order. They tend to perceive life crisis events of birth, marriage, death, illness, in the context of an extended local network of social support systems of kin and friends who provide emotional insurance and social meaning to these crises.

3. Children grow up conscious of the intergeneration family environment and their expectation of interdependency and reciprocal obligation is continuously reinforced.

4. The young person is socialized primarily in a community which is identified by the ancestral place, the language of the region (one of fourteen major languages), and by the family's social status which is usually derived from ancestral occupation and lineage.

5. Most college students are educated in or close to their home town under conditions where geographical mobility and the use of the automobile and the telephone is relatively infrequent.

6. Same sex friendships are very important in the growing up process and tend to be cultivated in depth and over time for long term permanence and fidelity (Amarasingham, 1980).

It is safe to generalize then that the typical graduate student from India — no matter how highly trained and academically qualified — comes to the United States with a strong sense of the family and friendship attachments that are part of his sense of identity and community. The psychosocial transition, thus, from the Indian physical and social milieu to the American campus environment represents a major discontinuity in life style and social role, and a disruption of natural support systems that validate his self-esteem.

The cross-cultural experience of study abroad then for the student whose normal socialization patterns are as described above represents a major environmental change and culture shock stresses for which new coping strategies are required

Culture shock is a sudden explosion of major environmental changes that are experienced in terms of loss in several respects.

(1) First, there is the culture shock of status loss. "I was somebody in my own society. I had love and respect from my friends and family back home; here I'm nobody, only a foreign student." Physical visibility may sensitize the student to his minority group status with attendant apprehensions about being slighted and discriminated against.

(2) Culture shock may also take the form of *uprooting of meaning* (Marris, 1980). Long and stable attachments to friends and family within a set of reciprocal obligations create a social texture of meaning in one's environment. Such friendship expectations and familial interdependencies are easily frustrated when one moves to a strange environment. Or they are not perceived to be meaningful or available in the American milieu. The result is a deep feeling of estrangement and loneliness. The trough of depression in the U-Curve may be interpreted in terms of such loss of meaning, which is compensated in great part by one's career purposes and immediate professional goals. The overcompensations are often costly.

(3) Culture shock may also be due to sensory overload and physiological fatigue that is experienced when environmental pressures accumulate and accentuate the academic demands. Individual variations need, of course, to be recognized within student groups in terms of capacity for stress tolerance or psychological "immunity" to the painful feelings of loss. This paper argues that students from developing societies which maintain more or less traditional family patterns of an early industrial civilization even in the large urban areas, may be much more vulnerable to emotional stress of loss than is usually recognized in orientation and counselling programs in American universities.

The serious mental health consequences of culture shock due to uprooting are illustrated in the following case materials reported by Coplan (1977).

A young artistic boy from a European country had recently moved to the United States following the father's most recent assignment in South America. At the time of referral, the boy was withdrawn in class and did not respond to anything. When the family moved to the U.S., not only was the boy's mother expecting another child, but for many weeks the whole family — including 8 children — had been living in hotels. All of this was in sharp contrast to the boy's experience in their South American home. There the family had a big house with servants and a leisurely life style. The boy had a private tutor to encourage his interest in art and the freedom to run to the mountains and streams near his home.

When he came to the U.S., he lost his special place in the family; he lost the freedom to run free, to cross the street, to develop his own pace. In a sense this boy had lost *everything* (from his point of view). He felt he was completely helpless, and he did not understand why his parents had to move or why he had lost these things. Therefore, he was always talking about running away. Fortunately at the school, there was an artistic teacher who was good at ceramics. The boy was enrolled in the program and that seemed to help . . .

The other case of culture shock was a bright young Nigerian girl who had rejoined her family members in the U.S. at the time of the Ibo war. She showed signs of hyperactivity and violence, and her high level of school achievement dropped. She was dismayed by her situation. Why could she not go out into the street to play? In Africa, she was used to going to the common pond, playing with other children. Here she found herself in a neighbourhood that was dangerous, where she was told not even to open a window. This girl had no structure of understanding to help her cope with the changes in her life. She eventually returned to her home country (Coplan, 1977).

It is noteworthy that recent major reviews of the comprehensive foreign student literature (Spaulding and Coelho, 1980) have noted the importance which foreign students attached to the role of co-nationals in guiding them through the early stages of culture shock. Thus, instant immersion in American culture as part of an orientation program may not be appropriate and may even be counter productive. The student may need to experience the ownership of his feelings of loss and of the attachments that have been the basis of his self-image and self-esteem and sense of community. These feelings of "mourning", as it were, have to be worked through, old attachments symbolically reconstituted over time to allow for new friendships to be developed. But these processes take time. Culture shock disturbances as noted above do not necessarily lead to pathological consequences, or "nervous breakdowns" in most students from developing societies. Nevertheless, we need focussed research to determine the nature and extent of the emotional stresses and their impacts on students in the high risk situations to which they are exposed in the course of study abroad through different stages of their sojourn.

A few practical suggestions may help to guide the programs of preventive maintenance of coping systems in foreign students especially from developing countries:

1. Counsellors should be trained in cross-cultural sensitivity such as in models developed by Pedersen (1978) or Triandis (1977).

2. Mental health specialists are least likely to be approached first, and may also be least accessible or appropriate, for the same reasons that Americans in trouble do not seek out psychiatrists at once.

3. These painful experiences of separation and loss, nostalgia and homesickness are not perceived by Indian students as illness or as mental health problems to be cured. In general, too, there is a fear of stigma that is attached to mental disturbance (Saran, 1980).

4. Cultural patterns in Latin America and Asia tend to emphasize the difficulties of life as pervasive human conditions, and the philosophic emphasis is on bearing up and containing the self (Cohen, 1980).

5. Friendly and knowledgeable tutors, wise counsellors, "gurus" who can give time and support on a one-to-one basis are likely to be accepted and effective in guiding the foreign student through the high risk situations of culture shock.

Research is needed: (a) to identify preparatory experiences that facilitate the psychosocial competence of students and the transfer of coping skills across cultural settings; (b) to describe and assess strategies of stress management in high risk situations during various phases of their sojourn from leaving home to re-entry into the home society. Selection and advisory personnel in the student's home country need to pay attention, as Klineberg (1980) has recommended, to the psychological qualities of students and their preparedness, or coping skills — at least as much as they now do to their academic qualifications and technical records on paper. Innovations in conceptual models and research methodologies are needed which focus on high risk situations faced by foreign students (especially from developing countries) during crucial phases of coping with stressful transitions in cross-cultural settings. We need new research knowledge which will help us understand:

(1) What factors in the student's situation at home and abroad determine the *various shapes of U-Curves* during the critical phases of adaptation to culture shock (e.g. the first year of the sojourn abroad as well as of the re-entry home)?

(2) What high risk group profiles characterize different shapes of U-Curves observed in different student population groups at these phases?

(3) What coping strategies are commonly used by foreign students in managing stressful high risk situations in various social and academic environments?

From such knowledge, evaluation criteria and program guidelines could be formulated for foreign student selection, training, orientation (in home and host country), placement, counselling, referral and follow-up support, etc., that would be useful to the students and their sponsors, as well as to practitioners and policy planners in International Educational and Cultural Exchange of persons.

In conclusion, it is suggested that research knowledge of high risk factors in stressful transition situations may have wide conceptual validity and practical utility for other student population groups which are exposed to culture shock in new environmental settings; for example, (a) minority group students from socially disadvantaged families in the U.S. or in developing countries, who are "first generational learners" in university settings; (b) American students, especially adolescents, whose re-entry in U.S. after having spent several years abroad with their families posted overseas, exposes them to culture shock stresses. As Spaulding and Coelho (1980) have suggested in a forthcoming volume which discusses issues of coping and adaptation in different kinds of cultural and environmental changes affecting uprooting populations,

... we know a great deal about what happens to foreign students in the United States, and how they are handled, and yet at the same time we know little ...

... many concerns of foreign students are similar to those of American students, thus suggesting that students have some common mental health problems related to culture goals no matter where they come from.

REFERENCES

Alexander, A. A. et al.
    1976 Psychotherapy and the foreign student. In: Pedersen, Lonner and Draguns (eds.), Counselling Across Cultures, University Press of Hawaii, Honolulu.

Amarasingham, L.
    1980 Making friends in a new culture: South Asian women in Boston. In: G. V. Coelho and P. Ahmed (eds.), Uprooting and Development. Plenum Publishers, New York.

Brislin, R. and Pedersen, P.
    1976 Cross-Cultural Orientation Programs. Gardner Press, New York.

Coelho, G. V. and Stein, J. J.
    1977 Coping with stresses of an urban planet: Impacts of uprooting and overcrowding. Habitat 2(3/4): 379–390.

Coelho, G. V. and Ahmed, P. (eds.)
    1980 Uprooting and Development. Plenum Publishers, New York.

Coelho, G. V., Hamburg, D. A. and Adams, J. E. (eds.)
    1974 Coping and Adaptation. Basic Books, New York.

Cohen, L.
    1980 Stress and coping among Latin American women immigrants. Ch. 16 in G. V. Coelho and P. Ahmed (eds.) op. cit.

Coplan, A.
    1977 Cross-cultural therapy. Presentation at the Washington International School and personal communication.

Klineberg, O.
    1980 Stressful experiences of foreign students at various stages of sojourn: Counselling and policy implications. Ch. 13 in G. V. Coelho and P. Ahmed (eds.) op. cit.

Lalonde, M.
    1974 A new perspective on the health of Canadians. Ministry of Health and Welfare, Ottawa, Canada.

Marris, P.
    1980 The uprooting of meaning. Ch. 5 in G. V. Coelho and P. Ahmed (eds.) op. cit.

Pedersen, P. B.
    1978 Counselling across cultures. Personnel and Guidance Journal, April.

Pedersen, P. B.
    1980 Role learning as a coping strategy. Ch. 14 in G. V. Coelho and P. Ahmed (eds.) op. cit.

Saran, P.
    1980 Social adaptation of Indian immigrants in the New York areas. Ch. 17 in G. V. Coelho and P. Ahmed (eds.) op. cit.

Spaulding, S. and Coelho, G. V.
    1980 Students from Abroad. Ch. 15 in G. V. Coelho and P. Ahmed (eds.) op. cit.

Triandis, H.
    1977 Interpersonal Behavior. Brooks Cole, Monterey, California.

White, R. H.
    1974 Strategies of adaptation. Ch. 4 in G. V. Coelho, D. A. Hamburg and J. E. Adams (eds.) op. cit.

World Health Organization
    1979 Psychosocial factors and health. Ch. 5 in P. I. Ahmed and G. V. Coelho (eds.) Toward a New Definition of Health: Psychosocial Dimensions, Plenum Publishers, New York.

AKIRA HOSHINO, Ph.D.

AN ELABORATION OF THE "CULTURE-SHOCK" PHENOMENON: ADJUSTMENT PROBLEMS OF JAPANESE YOUTH RETURNING FROM OVERSEAS

Dr. Coelho's excellent paper deals with a matter about which I have much interest. I refer specifically to what has been described as a "double uprooting" process.

For several years, I have been interested in the problems of "returnees", children of Japanese parents who have been working overseas and then returning to Japan. These young people are somewhat different from college students spending several years in the U.S. because these children have not left Japan by their own free will for a specific purpose, as in the case of exchange students.

After the 1960's, with the rapid expansion of Japanese industries and internationalization of the Japanese economy, at least 3,000 Japanese companies opened branch offices or joint offices in foreign countries. Employees were sent to these countries to work in the foreign offices. At first, the children were left behind but eventually their families were brought to join them. It is these children who face the problems as the "returnees".

These are not only sons and daughters of bankers and electronics engineers, camera, or auto company workers but of many varied types of inductries. In New York City alone, at least 5,000–6,000 Japanese are working and living with their families. This trend is rising in all the major cities of the world.

The parents have three major decisions regarding their children when working in these foreign environments: (1) Do they trust the schools in the area in which they are working? Or (2) Should the children remain in Japan with their grandparents or relatives for their education? And (3) If they do find good schools in their new locations, should the children attend "international schools" or go to the local school?

In the United States, Britain, France, or Germany, there is a trend to send the children to public schools, but parents are more hesitant to do this in developing countries. As a result of this problem, parents have pressured the Japanese government for Japanese schools within these countries. Since 1975, there are more than ten Japanese schools in foreign countries for the express purpose of helping the Japanese children to retain their Japanese cultural identity. Despite the emergence of these schools, three problems have remained with these children:

1. The school system in Japan is of a very high standard and is geared for the high competition for college entrance. This factor causes parents to worry about the caliber of their children's education in the foreign countries, and whether or not the children will be able to get into the elite, high status universities in Japan they would like them to attend.

2. The second problem is the diversity of views and ways of thinking

specifically in personal relationships) between the Japanese and the views held in other cultures.

3. The third problem is the discrimination and prejudice held by the Japanese natives against the returning Japanese children from other cultures. Japan, as a country, has been monocultural and mono-lingual. It is hard for native Japanese to relate to those Japanese children who, though they physically appear the same, return home with different views and values. These children are neither immigrants nor of an ethnic or political minority, and yet they are thorns in the side of the native group. Teachers may ignore these children, or may single them out as bad examples. In some cases, teachers may even show some antagonism towards these students. The Minister of Education and many teachers in the Japanese school system are now realizing that the problem will become more serious unless more effort is made to integrate the returning Japanese children back into their own culture.

Last Spring, the International Christian University in Tokyo, which was established about 30 years ago, opened another branch, an international school called ICU high school. Among the 300—400 students attending, two-thirds are "returnees", and the remainder are from local Japanese schools.

We are now doing research to follow up these students' adjustment back into the school, and looking for ways to make this process more successful. Aside from this research at the college level, I have met with many returning students, including some maladjusted and pathological cases. One of my graduate students has written a thesis on these students. In our studies we have found that three key factors are involved in the individual adjustment processes: (1) Does the student have a goal or a concrete purpose in life? (2) Does the student have family ties? And (3) Does the student identify as a Japanese? If a student has all of these factors, there is not much to worry about in their adjustment potential. However, a student without these factors will encounter difficulty. For instance, a Japanese student returning from five or six years in the United States to a school in Japan will have difficulty coping with Japanese life, and with Japanese friends on campus. They are now "Japanese-Americans", and usually would prefer to return to the United States.

In one extreme example, a few years ago we encountered a female student with acute psychotic symptoms as a result of the "returnee" problem. On our campus, we felt inadequate to meet her needs as we are without facilities to cope with psychiatric problems of adjustment. This illustrated to us our urgent need to face this problem on a general level as well as in specific cases such as hers. Teachers and mental health workers must be made aware of this adjustment problem as well as the need to find solutions.

ALI NAHIT BABAOGLU, M.D.

SOME SOCIAL AND PSYCHIATRIC ASPECTS OF UPROOTING AMONG TURKISH IMMIGRANT WORKERS IN WEST GERMANY

Foreign workers in advanced industrialized European countries represent a special kind of migration. These worker migrants do not move with the intention of settling in the host countries. They plan to return to their own homelands someday and, therefore, they tend to maintain strong connections with the home country. In the meanwhile, these millions of foreign workers in Europe often represent a great social problem within the receiving countries. The solutions offered are mostly directed to the social, economical, and cultural assimilation of these masses. However, the assimilation of the foreign worker often means changing a sociological problem of the "hosts" to a psychological problem of the "guests".

In this paper, the social and psychiatric aspects of Turkish workers in West Germany are examined. This group of foreign workers is of interest because they exhibit characteristics which seem to run contrary to some general assumptions about the migrant worker in Europe. Since 1972, Turkish workers comprise the largest single group among all of the foreign workers in West Germany. Despite an economic recession in the late 1970's, which saw nearly 100,000 return home to Turkey, the Turkish foreign workers still number over 500,000; and together with their families, they reach a total number of over one and a half million.

SOME DEMOGRAPHIC CHARACTERISTICS

It is well known that in many respects, the demographic characteristics of foreign workers are different from the populations of both the home and host countries. For example, the proportionate number in the productive ages is much higher among the migrant workers, with the result that their common illness rate is lower and the birth rate higher. If we take a closer look at the demographic data, we can see some further characteristics which carry serious implications for the social and psychological health of the workers. A good example is found in statistics on their marriage and home status.

Taken as a total group, most of the foreign workers in West Germany are married. However, there are some differences among the various ethnic groups: Italians show the lowest rate of married men; Yugoslavs have the lowest rate of married women. On the other hand, the Turks have one of the highest rates of both married men and women. This picture, however, must also consider the number of married workers who live in West Germany without their partners. Here, the lowest rate among married men is found in the Greeks, followed by the Spaniards and the Italians. At the other extreme, 2/3 of Turkish, and 1/2 of

Yugoslav married men are away from their wives. These figures are well above the average of about 40 percent of all married male workers whose spouses are absent. The trends among married females from Turkey and Yugoslavia are about the same. Taking all married female workers together, about 10 percent do not have their husbands with them. But against this overall average, nearly 1/5 of Yugoslav, and more than 1/4 of Turkish married women are living in West Germany far from their husbands and families.

It is generally known that immigration and foreign worker migration flow from unindustrialized societies to industrialized ones; and it is a fact that most of the foreign workers in Europe come from the under-developed regions of their home countries. However, the Turkish workers again show a pattern wihich is reversed. The most under-developed regions of Turkey are the eastern, south-eastern, and north-eastern areas of Anatolia, and the highly-developed ones are the Marmar, Aegean, and Mediterranean regions. In contrast to the general pattern of other worker-exporting countries, the greatest proportion of Turkish migrant workers (56%) come from the highly developed regions of Turkey, according to the records of the Turkish Ministry of Labor. A comparison of the applications to the Turkish Labour offices in 8 provinces with higher, and 8 provinces with lower, worker-export rates, shows that workers in the under-developed eastern regions have very little interest to go abroad.

This pattern is supported by a comparison among several migrant worker nationalities in West Germany, according to their place of last establishment (village, town, or city). Among Greeks and Spaniards, about 70% came from villages and rural areas. Among the Italians, the rate is about 60%. Only 12% to 21% of the workers from these three countries were citizens of large cities before they came to Germany. In contrast, about 40% of the Turkish workers in Germany came from large cities (over 100,000 population); about 35% from towns (between 5,000 and 100,000 population); and just 25% came from rural areas and villages.

There are some further interesting features among the Turkish workers in West Germany. Some 82% of the men, and 21% of the women had a regular job before they went abroad (corresponding figures for the Greek workers, for example, were 64% for males and 18% for females). Turkish workers have been among the highest skilled of all migrant worker groups in West Germany. In 1972, about 55% of the Turkish workers were considered to be at a highly skilled level (Italians were 48%, and Greeks were 44%). These figures indicate that labor importing countries want skilled and semi-skilled people who do not require much in the way of social investments such as education and training. One effect of this policy is that Turkish women workers in West Germany have a much higher education level than the average woman in Turkey. (In West Germany, 35% of Turkish women have high school graduation, and 88% have at lest 5 years of formal schooling).

Another characteristic of the Turkish workers is that of a previous move within Turkey. Nearly 70% were born elsewhere from their place of last residence prior to their going abroad to West Germany. The majority of Turks seem to be undergoing a social promotion process, even within Turkey itself. The aim is to elevate one's social status in order to secure a higher position in the middle-class structure. These life goals are reflected in the following responses given by Turkish workers, when asked about their motivations for going to West Germany: To get a greater amount of money quickly; to secure the future of the family; to get better professional skills; and to obtain better educational opportunities for their children.

Almost all of the workers (95%) want to go back to Turkey eventually. About three-quarters want to settle in a large city after they return. No more than 7% are satisfied with being an industrial worker, and only 6% wish to become farmers. Only 3% of the Turkish workers have no particular idea or plan about their future; and 80% invest regularly in Turkey from their savings.

SOME PSYCHIATRIC ASPECTS

There is a general awareness that the first year or so following migration is the most critical. The uprooting experience, and the early difficulties in a new society can often lead to depression and breakdown. Because of the lack of verbal contact due to language differences, the depression is often expressed through psychosomatic disturbances. But all of the anxiety reactions, depression, and psychosomatic disorders during the early months of settlement may hide more serious illnesses. The remaining part of this paper examines some psychiatric cases involving Turks who were seen in a psychiatric hospital in West Germany over a period of 12 years. The hospital is the Rheinisches Landeskrankenhaus Duren, a public service hospital in Duren, a middle-to-large town located between Aachen and Koln.

From 1965 until 1977, a total of 157 admissions of persons from Turkish origin came to this hospital. Some of the cases are repeat admissions, however, and the actual number of unduplicated cases is 125 persons. Of this number, 95 are studied from their case records; the remaining 30 are patients personally seen by the writer. Following admission, 10 of the patients were diagnosed as purely neurological cases. The other 115 cases were mentally ill (21 women and 94 men). Of these, 90 were hospitalized only once; the others came twice or more. The most important social-psychological data on the 115 mentally ill patients are given in the following summary:

Age: Most of the patients were between 12 and 35 years of age. Only one man was over fifty years of age; and 5 women and 4 men were younger than twenty.

Marriage: Most of the patients were married, although many did not have their partners with them in West Germany. Only 3 women patients and 34 men were not married; 3 women and 7 men were widowed, or separated. Of the 68 married cases, 14 women and 15 men were together with their spouses.

Education: There were no records on the educational background of 44 patients. Of the others, 3 women and one man had no formal education; 8 women and 11 men had less than eight years of education; and 4 women and 44 men had an education exceeding eight years.

Birthplace and Last Turkish Residence: The region of origin is not known in 29 cases. Of the others, 40 of the patients were from the western region of Turkey; 25 were from the middle region; and 19 from the eastern parts. Only two of the patients were born outside of Turkey. The last place of residence in Turkey is not known in 23 of the cases. Of the others, 49 were from rural areas, and 43 from urban areas. Among the latter, 22 patients from a city background had a previous experience in migration within Turkey.

Occupation in Turkey: There is no information here for 35 patients. The employment backgrounds of the others were as follows: Industrial worker (22); Housewife (15); Farmer (14); Artisan (10); Student (6); Technical Personnel (4); Policeman and Watchman (4); Without Work (4); Under Aged (1).

Time in Germany at First Admission: Among those with an earlier history of psychiatric disturbances, 13 cases out of 24 (54%) were admitted into the hospital during their first 18 months in West Germany. In contrast to this, 19 cases out of 91 (20%) were patients without any known history of psychiatric disturbance who were hospitalized during their first 18 months abroad. Interestingly, this picture is reversed among those patients who had been in West Germany for over 5 years. Of this group, 5 patients had a history of mental illness; but there were 24 patients who did not have any known previous disorders.

Premorbid Predisposition: As noted earlier, 24 of the 115 cases had a previous history of psychiatric disturbance. However, our designation of "predisposed" cases also included other kinds of situations, sometimes of a questionable nature. For example, a patient with a low schooling level who comes from a family where other members are highly educated was counted as "predisposed". Taking these into account, the number of patients with any kind of premorbid predisposition was 40.

Healing: Taking into account the previous 40 cases as predisposed, the treatment record of all the patients is given in the Table 1, where very different trends are shown by the 2 categories of cases:

TABLE I
Treatment Record

Healing	Predisposed	Not predisposed	Total
Within 5 days	3	32	35
Between 5–10 days	7	14	21
Between 10–20 days	6	9	15
Between 20–30 days	5	9	14
More than 30 days	5	5	10
Not healed	14	6	20
Total	40	75	115

Relationship to the Environment: This category was an attempt to assess a patient's social connections with Germany and Turkey. Unfortunately, information was classified under some very gross headings, and some social data of a subjective type were interpreted very arbitrarily. Keeping these things in mind, Table II gives an impression of the social relations of the patients. The numbers do not add up to 100% because the same patient may be counted in more than one category:

TABLE II
Relationship to Environment

	Predisposed	Not predisposed	Total
Isolation from Turks	10	12	22
Rupture from Turkey	8	11	19
Struggle with Turks	9	16	25
Friendship to Germans	9	23	32
Sex-relation with Germans	8	6	14
Severe moral-change in Germany	11	7	18
Subjective identification to Germans	7	16	23
Strong signs of assimilation	12	44	56

Clinical Diagnoses: Some 49 of the patients were diagnosed as "paranoid hallucinatory psychoses in schizophrenia group". Among these, 21 were categorized as predisposed cases. Another 29 patients were diagnosed as "depressive or reactive depressive reaction or psychosis". Among these were 4 predisposed cases. As mentioned earlier, a number of the cases were seen personally by this writer, and these diagnoses were classified a little differently: 6 patients showed a short-term psychotic reaction which was healed spontaneously within 48 hours; 8 patients had a longer termed schizophrenic psychosis; 2 patients were seen in an acute manic state; 8 cases had short-termed reactive depressive states; 3 had hypochondriac complaints with evidently depressive features. And one was a case of a murderer who was described in court as "psychotic". In summarizing the information on these patients, the tables at the end of this paper categorize the various kinds of data under 4 groups of diagnoses: Group I is Short-term psychotic states; Group II is Progressive-psychotic delusion systems; Group III is Reactive-depressive states; and Group IV is an "Other" category which subsumes such items as MDP and Alcoholism.

SUMMARY

A great proportion of Turkish workers in West Germany seem to have the ability and tendency to become adapted and integrated into German social life. This may be due to the fact that the Turkish workers who go abroad tend to be a group which is relatively well-educated and better skilled. These workers have ambitions of socially elevating themselves and their families, and to secure a higher social status position. This is more likely to occur if the workers eventually return home to Turkey where they are not considered as outsiders. However, these workers are under tremendous pressure to assimilate into West German society. For them, to be assimilated means to give up their hope of winning a higher social place in a Turkish society where they are totally accepted, and to be satisfied with a lower social place in a West Germany society. Because of this conflict, we must be concerned about its possible effects upon the social and psychological health of the Turkish migrant workers.

TABLE III
Summary Data on Social and Diagnostic Categories

	GROUP I Short-term Psychotic States	GROUP II Progressive- Psychotic Delusion Systems	GROUP III Reactive- Depressive States	GROUP IV Other	TOTAL
Number (a) Male	42	21	25	6	94
(b) Female	5	–	15	1	21
Age (a) below 20	3	2	4	1	10
(b) between 20 and 30	30	6	14	5	55
(c) between 31 and 40	12	9	20	1	42
(d) between 41 and 50	2	3	2	–	7
(e) Over 50	–	1	–	–	1
Marriage (a) Single	19	6	9	3	37
(b) Married together with partner	13	4	15	1	33
(c) Married, alone	14	10	11	2	37
(d) Widow, separated	1	1	5	1	8

TABLE III (continued).

Residence in Turkey					
(a) Rural area	27	14	14	5	60
(b) Urban area	12	4	16	–	32
(c) Unknown	8	3	10	2	23
Mental Disorder Before	9	11	3	1	24
Premorbid Predisposition	7	4	3	2	16
Duration of residence in Germany					
(a) Below 1 year	10	2	3	–	15
(b) Between 1–3 years	22	10	13	2	21
(c) Between 3–5 years	7	4	8	2	21
(d) Between 5–8 years	6	2	10	1	19
(e) Over 8 years	2	3	6	1	12
Healing by first admission					
(a) Within 5 days	24	–	7	4	35
(b) 5–10 days	8	–	13	–	21
(c) 10–20 days	5	2	7	1	15
(d) Over 20 days	7	4	12	1	24
(e) No healing	3	15	1	1	20
Admission number: 1	34	13	38	5	90
2	10	4	1	1	16
3	2	1	1	1	5
More	1	3	–	–	4

TABLE IV
Summary Data on Clinical and Diagnostic Categories

	GROUP I Short-term Psychotic States	GROUP II Progressive- Psychotic Delusion Systems	GROUP III Reactive- Depressive States	GROUP IV Other	TOTAL
Clinical Picture					
(a) Murder and attempt	1	4	1	–	6
(b) Suicide and attempt	2	1	11	–	14
(c) Aggression	15	3	2	1	21
(d) Disturbed memory	8	1	2	1	12
(e) Fear	14	3	4	1	22
(f) Sorrow, mourning	31	6	40	5	82
(g) Persecution against Turks	18	11	–	–	29
(h) Persecution against Germans	2	3	–	1	6
(i) Political persecutive delusions	13	6	–	–	19
(j) Religious delusions, ideas	13	4	16	2	35
(k) Impotence	–	–	2	–	2
(l) Hypochondriac ideas	3	4	15	1	23

TABLE IV (continued).

Relation to the environment					
(a) Isolation from Turks	5	7	8	2	22
(b) Rupture from Turkey	8	5	4	2	19
(c) Struggle with Turks	9	5	9	2	25
(d) Good contact to German	14	5	10	3	32
(e) German Girl/Boy Friend	4	4	5	1	14

REFERENCES

Abadan-Unat, N.
    1977 Goc ve Gelisme, Ankara Universitesi, Ankara.
Becker, R. et al.
    Fremdarbeiterbeschaftigung in deutschen Kapitalismus. Das Argument 68: 741–756.
Benkert, H. et al.
    1974 Psychische Storungen bei ausl. Arbeitnehmern, Der Nervenarzt 45: 76–87.
Boker, W.
    1975 Psychiatrie der Gastarbeiter. In: Psychiatrie der Gegenwert, Vol. III, Springer Wurzburg: 429–466.
Castles and Kosack
    1973 Immigrant Workers and Class Structure in Western Europe. Oxford Univ. Press, London.
Friessem, D. H.
    1974 Psych. und Psychosomatische Erkrankungen Ausl. Arbeitnehmer. Psychiat. Neurol. med. Psychol, Leipzig 26: 78–90.
Klee, E.
    1975 Gastarbeiter. Suhrkamp, Frankfurt.
Mehrlander, U.
    1974 Soziale Aspekte der Auslanderbeschaftigung. Neue Gesellschaft, Bonn.
Turkish Ministry of Foreign Affairs
    1976 Migration Movements Abroad. Department of Citizenship, Ankara.
Zwingmann, C. A. and Pfister-Ammende, M.
    1973 Uprooting and After. Springer-Verlag, New York.

MORTON BEISER, M.D.

MIGRATION IN A DEVELOPING COUNTRY: RISK AND OPPORTUNITY*

Migration from countryside to city, a ubiquitous Third World Phenomenon, involves not only physical change, but demands rapid accommodation to new cultural forms. It is usually assumed that migrants exposed to these demands become overwhelmed by stress, paying the price for modernization by developing physical and psychosomatic illnesses. A commonly held and popular notion, this assumption has also been enshrined in the behavioural sciences literature under the rubric, "the acculturative stress hypothesis". In its simplest form, this hypothesis assumes a form something like: "Rapid social change creates a condition of risk and the health of persons exposed to such change can be expected to suffer". Despite its continuing popularity, the acculturative stress formulation can no longer be considered tenable, at least in this simplistic form. Research results refute the hypothesis at least as often as they support it. (See for example, Alfred, 1965; De Vos & Miner, 1959; Fried, 1964; Gampel *et al.*, 1962; Graves, 1973; Murphy, 1977; Senghor, 1969; Scotch, 1963 as studies which support the hypothesis; Beiser & Collomb, 1981; Beiser *et al.*, 1976; Inkeles & Smith, 1974, 1976 as studies which refute it.)

There are probably several explanations for the discrepant findings yielded in the migration and social change literatures. One is that the model, "Social change is bad for mental health" does not take into account the complexities of real situations. In a state of flux, contingencies exist which modify the exigencies of change and which, in turn, affect health outcomes. Another problem is that insufficient attention has been paid to the question of change from what to what? In much of the research carried out in Africa, for example, cities are considered the crucible of change; villages in the "bush" are portrayed, by contrast, as utopias of stability and tradition (Inkeles & Smith, 1974). A growing body of findings, demonstrating that urban migrants fail to develop worse mental health than people in rural areas, suggests that either city environments are less maleficent than one would have thought, or that the countryside is a less benign setting than it is often imagined to be. In industrializing countries, both rural and urban areas are changing. The few rural-based mental health studies from Africa (Assael & German, 1970; Leighton *et al.*, 1963; Murphy, 1973) demonstrate that heterogeneity, rather than uniformity, characterizes these environments and that the effects on mental health are complex.

In Senegal, West Africa, both city and countryside are being transformed; in both settings, change creates conditions of risk and of opportunity. The current study is concerned with the Serer, of Senegal, West Africa. In the epidemiological portion of the study, we compare the health and mental health of rural Serer who have migrated to Dakar with Serer who have remained in their traditional, pastoral villages. Case studies of individual urban migrants examine the process of successful coping exemplified by some of the urban migrants, as well as the health consequences experienced by others who fail to adapt to changing circumstances. Case studies of villages are utilized to demonstrate that the rural environment is also changing, and that the type and rate of change occurring in a rural environment affect mental health.

SETTING OF THE STUDY

Since 1960, when it gained independence from France, Senegal has grown to a nation of 4 million people governed on the model of a European republic. Lacking natural resources or an industrial base of any significance, most Senegalese maintain themselves by subsistence farming and fishing. Rice and peanuts make up the only cash crops.

The Serer of Senegal, numbering about 600,000, remain one of the most traditional peoples in West Africa. While their origins are obscure, the weight of evidence suggests that their peace-loving ancestors were routed by warlike neighbours from Mali during the Mandinke reign of the 13th and 14th centuries. Approximately 600 years ago, a subgroup of the Serer settled in Niakhar, part of the Sine-Saloum, an arid territory of sand and scrub brush which permits little more than a lean subsistence. Here the Serer raise some livestock and, during a three-month rainy season, grow grain and peanuts. Because access to the region is difficult, and because over the past 600 years there has been little here to attract others to plunder, the Serer have remained an isolated, traditional people (See Figure 1) As recently as the early 1960s, Reverdy, the French anthropologist, called the region a "museum of Serer culture" (Reverdy, 1963). Features of the culture include ancestor and spirit worship, a bilateral kinship system, and castes. Religion, kinship and caste continue to shape much of the life of the villages — who speaks with the most authority, who will have access to which goods and which lands, and who can marry whom. (See also Delpech, 1967; Gamble, 1967; Reverdy, 1963.)

At least two major forces are now transforming this cultural museum. The first of these forces, the village cooperative movement, was introduced by the Ministry of Development and Rural Expansion of the new Senegalese Republic as part of the national goal of promoting "African Socialism" (Former President Dia as quoted in the U.N., 1964.) Under the plan, the Ministry divided all the villages in the Sine into groups of three, each such group constituting a cooperative. Rather than marketing their peanuts as a family group, Serer peasants who join the cooperative now bring their produce to the Secco — a centralized collecting agency in one of the villages; the cooperative negotiates prices and arranges for transport. Through the cooperative, the Serer can obtain advance credit for a maximum of 25% the value of their previous year's crop in order to buy seeds, fertilizer and farm implements. An elected management council, with representatives from each of the villages, administers the cooperative and

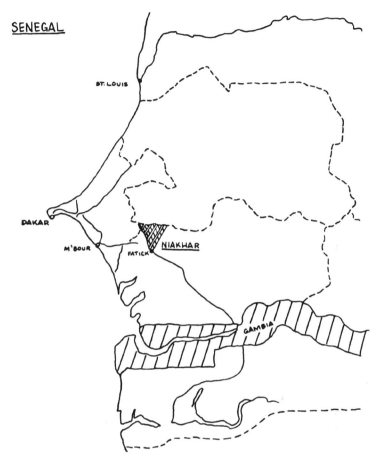

Fig. 1.

reports to a regional representative of the Ministry of Development and Rural Expansion. While the explicit goal of the cooperative movement is efficient management and marketing, the underlying thrust is to redistribute power. The cooperatives replace the feudalistic system of inherited property and power and the caste system of inherited social status with a social order which stresses individual achievement and a balancing of power through a system of elected representatives.

The plan threatens tradition in a number of ways. It displaces the authority of the council of elders — a village chief and chiefs of extended family units, all of whom assume their titles through inheritance — in favor of a supra-village authority, members of which will be elected (or, more probably, appointed by government representatives). Individual achievement, which determines election to a management position, is antithetical to Serer values which stress the submerging of the individual to collective groups such as family, clan, and village. Common ownership of land and of major pieces of equipment is, in many ways, even more threatening since the entire religious and social system of the Serer is predicated upon the transmission of property from an ancestor to his descendants. The government has abolished the hereditary monarchy of the Sine and threatens to overthrow the whole system of property ownership. For the time being, people can continue to work inherited lands; however, any lands which lie fallow revert to government claim. Another obstacle to the acceptance of the cooperatives stems from the fact that the Federal Ministry, interested mainly in what makes economic sense, decides which combination of three villages will make up a cooperative. What the economic planners overlook are cultural forces which sometimes make their groupings impossible. Some villages, for instance, have refused to form a cooperative because of traditional rivalries, other because no recognized social relationships exist which would legitimize such an activity. Even though the villages which adopt the cooperative model experience demonstrable economic advantage, acceptance in the Sine continues to be uneven (Reverdy, 1963; U.N., 1964).

Overpopulation constitutes a second major threat to tradition. While the Sine has been densely populated for many years, overgrazing, overutilization of the land, and a severe drought which occurred in the early 1970s, together with a population increase due to improvements in health care, have combined to create a situation where the needs of the villagers overtax what their fields can provide them. Migration, based on the hope of finding work in cities like Dakar, has become the major response to this crisis (Rémy, 1974; Reverdy, 1963; WHO, 1960).

In Dakar, Serer are exposed to major forces of change — a dominant population of Wolof whose traditions are often at variance with those of the Serer; a population of 30,000 Europeans; Islam, the most powerful opponent of Serer animistic religion; a European and Middle-eastern dominated economy; evidences of western material culture such as automobiles, electrical appliances, movies, sophisticated restaurants and discotheques.

Serer from the Sine locate in five neighbourhoods in Dakar. Three of these are transitional areas, the other two more permanent suburbs. In the transitional areas, many Serer, women in particular, remain segrated from their Wolof, Faluni, and European neighbours and village ties exert the most significant influence on their lives. They have been chosen to come to Dakar in order to help support their families in the village, and their first allegiance continues to be to the Sine. A formal Serer organization, "Le Sine", exerts a strong influence in the transitional areas, offering financial assistance to newcomers and also serving in various ways to preserve ties between city and bush. Most Serer from Niakhar who live in Dakar are reluctant to say they have migrated, clinging instead to a goal of returning to the bush. When a young woman marries, she will leave Dakar to go to live with her husband's father's family. A young man will have longer to wait. He remains in the city until he has earned enough money so that his family's lack of land no longer poses a hardship — or until his place can be taken by someone else.

Some Serer have, however, moved from the transitional zones to more permanent neighbourhoods, the new suburbs of Dakar. Rather than sending their wives back to their father's village, suburban Serer — the first generation of permanent migrants — live in Dakar with their wives and children.

METHODS OF THE STUDY

A. *Selection of Samples*

The region of Niakhar, in the Sine-Saloum, the area where we chose to do our rural survey, has a population of 35,187 (according to a 1965 government census). These people live in 65 different villages with a median size of 300. Two principal aims dictated the selection of a rural sample: (1) in order to make rural-urban comparisons possible, the sample would have to be representative of adults living in the region of Niakhar, and (2) in order to permit analyses to be carried out of interactions between differing sociocultural environments and health, the sample would have to be stratified so as to assure a range of different types of villages in the region. The sampling task was made easier because the results of a government survey of Niakhar which had been carried out several years earlier, were made available to our research team. From a total of several hundred items which the survey covered, we selected 29 social, demographic, and economic variables: the basis of selection was that a significant number of subjects had responded to an item and that it possessed potential theoretical interest. These 29 variables were subjected to a principal components factor analysis followed by varimax rotation. The three factors which emerged, together accounting for 58.5% of total item variance, have been labelled Modernity, Exposure and Instability.

Villages scoring high on Modernity show evidence of having adopted the cooperative system; they have established patterns of credit; they tend to be prospering economically; Islam has begun to make inroads against the traditional, animistic religion; on a proportional basis, there are relatively few elderly men who live here as compared with villages low on Modernity. Villages high on Exposure are ethnically heterogeneous, with Wolof as well as Serer inhabitants; they are located near principal roads and there are various kinds of public access. Villages high on Instability are characterized by a great deal of in-and-out migration and tend to have smaller family units living together within them.

By assigning scores of high, medium, and low on the first factor, and high and low on each of the remaining two, we created 12 typologies (3 × 2 × 2). Each village could be assigned to one, and only one of these types, and, using a table of random numbers, we then selected one village from each group to be representative of that type. We next conducted a census of all family compounds within the sample villages and of adults living within the compounds. Since we wished to obtain a total sample of 300, we divided the total population of each village by 25 in order to give a sampling interval (for example, a village with 300 adults would have an interval of 12; every 12th person enumerated would be chosen for the sample). We used a table of random numbers to determine which number between 0 and 9 would be the point of entry into each village and then drew the sample. The technique in some respects was a modification of Kish's method for sampling urban areas with village compounds taking the place of city blocks (Kish, 1965) and also resembles Tryon's social area analyses (Tryon, 1955). (The study was designed to deal with adults. It is very difficult to establish precise ages with the Serer, and it is doubly difficult to know what to consider a suitable cutting point for an "adult". For example, girls begin to marry and to bear children at 12 and 13. Therefore, although we attempted to limit the sample to people 15 or older, the precise age breakdown is questionable.) With the study already underway, the chief of one of the villages — a village we had reason to suspect was in the throes of considerable social upheaval — forbade any further participation. At this point, it proved impossible to substitute another village of the same type. After refusals and other attrition, the sample size attained was 269, and interview data were collected on 236 people. Comparison of age and sex distributions of the sample with population figures for the entire region did not reveal any gross sampling distortions.

Field workers lived in each of the eleven sample villages for at least one month in order to develop ethnographic descriptions and in order to prepare the villages for the interviews which were to follow. Their descriptions confirm the meaningfulness of the typologies constructed on the basis of our nomothetic approach.

An age and sex breakdown of the rural sample appears in Table I.

TABLE I
Rural Sample: Age and Sex Distribution

Age	Male	Female	Total	Per Cent
10–19	12	14	26	11.0
20–29	15	22	37	15.7
30–39	16	35	51	21.6
40–49	22	33	55	23.3
50–59	15	20	35	14.8
60–69	11	5	16	6.8
70+	8	8	16	6.8
Total	99	137	236	100.0
Per cent	41.9	58.1		

A total census of Serer from Niakhar living in Dakar yielded a list of 807 names (the best estimate is that for each two names gathered in this way, there are nine people who fail to be enumerated) (Beiser and Collomb, 1981). We attempted to draw a probability sample of 300 subjects from this urban census. Because of attrition, due mainly to migration after the completion of the census, and several cases of refusal, our sample dropped to 269. Among these, 220 urban migrants responded to the psychiatric questionnaire. Forty percent of the total census were young women under 20. Since strictly random sampling would have resulted in a preponderance of these people, we sampled women under 20 at a rate of one in four, while everyone else was sampled at a rate of one in two. The age and sex breakdown of the sample is described in Table II.

TABLE II
Urban Sample: Age and Sex Distribution

Age	Male	Female	Total	Per Cent
10–19	21	39	60	27.3
20–29	57	29	86	39.1
30–39	28	14	42	19.1
40–49	13	11	24	10.1
50–59	3	2	5	2.3
60–69	2	1	3	1.4
70+	0	0	0	0
Total	124	96	220	100.0
Per cent	56.4	43.6		

The urban sample is strikingly skewed toward the younger ages. Migration is a relatively recent phenomenon, primarily involving the young; the result is that there are almost no Serer in Dakar over the age of 50. Slightly more than 50 percent of the urban sample are illiterate, 90 percent of the rural people can neither read, write, nor speak French. In the analyses, we adjusted for the underrepresentation of urban females under 20, for the differences in the size of the population falling into the different village strata, and for the respective sizes of the referent populations from which the urban and rural samples were drawn.

B. *Examination of the Sample Respondents*

Field work for the epidemiological study took place between March and July, 1970. Each subject was seen on three occasions. During the first contact, Serer-speaking, trained interviewers administered an interview schedule containing questions which elicited basic social and demographic data as well as questions which tapped a broad range of the respondents' attitudes, their views of the world, and their adherence to traditional or modern ways.

During the second contact, senior medical students and faculty from the University of Dakar Medical School conducted medical examinations. Each subject was asked to respond to a medical history and received a physical examination which included height and weight, a chest x-ray, hemoglobin and hematocrit, urinalysis, VDRL, stool and blood smear examination for parasites, and serum determinations for levels of cholesterol, glucose, urea, albumin, and transaminase. Specialists in dentistry, dermatology and ophthamology examined each subject and their reports became part of the total medical dossier. Blood pressure readings, obtained in a standardized fashion, constitute one of the dependent variables examined in this report.

The mental health questionnaire was administered during the third contact. The manner in which this instrument was developed has been described elsewhere (see Beiser *et al.*, 1976). Using factor analysis, we constructed four scales called Physiological Anxiety, Topical Depression, Health Preoccupation and Episodic Anxiety. These scales demonstrate concurrent and construct validity, a topic which forms the basis for a report which has appeared elsewhere (see scales, with item loadings as they appeared in the original factor analyses in Table III through VI. See also Beiser *et al.*, 1976).

TABLE III
Scale I (Physiological Anxiety)

Item	Original Factor Loading
1. Does your head feel heavy?	.564
2. Are you ever bothered by your hands being sweaty and clammy?	.557
3. Have you ever been troubled with constipation?	.536
4. Does your food ever seem tasteless and hard to swallow?	.534
5. Do your hands ever tremble enough to bother you?	.502
6. Do you ever have a sense of pressure in your head?	.477
7. Do you ever have loss of appetite?	.463
8. Do you have hemorrhoids?	.448
9. Have you ever had spells of dizziness?	.438
10. Do your arms and legs go to sleep rather easily?	.390
11. Are you ever bothered by nightmares?	.379
12. Do you take medicine for constipation?	.374
13. Are you ever troubled by upset stomach?	.365
14. Have you ever been bothered by your heart beating hard?	.359
15. Do you ever have creeping feelings in the skin?	.305
16. Are you ever troubled by a feeling that your hair is standing on end?	.360

TABLE IV
Scale II (Topical Depression)

Item	Original Factor Loading
1. Do you worry about what people say about you?	.555
2. Do you ever get so wrapped up in something you don't know what is going on around you?	.519
3. Are you easily distracted?	.508
4. Have you ever had to go easy on work?	.501
5. Do you feel weak all over much of the time?	.479
6. Are there times when you feel low or hopeless?	.478
7. Do you worry about money?	.461
8. Do you worry about family problems?	.443
9. Have there been times when you lost interest in everything?	.429
10. Do you feel you are an unlucky person?	.426
11. Do you sometimes worry for no reason?	.420
12. Do you ever feel that for no apparent reason people pick quarrels with you?	.406
13. Do you get angry?	.373
14. Do you sometimes wonder if anything is worthwhile any more?	.364
15. Do you have trouble making up you mind?	.326

TABLE V
Scale III (Health Preoccupation)

Item	Original Factor Loading
1. How is your health?	.641
2. Is your health in general all right?	.628
3. Do you worry about your physical health?	.511
4. Do you have any worries about your health?	.490
5. Do you have any troubles with your joints?	.483
6. Do you have kidney trouble?	.433
7. Do you wake up easily at night?	.416
8. Are you often tired when you wake up in the morning?	.410
9. Do you have back trouble?	.364
10. Do you have trouble seeing?	.303

TABLE VI
Scale IV (Episodic Anxiety)

Item	Original Factor Loading
Are you easily upset?	.475
If yes:	
When you are upset:	
1. Do you have palpitations?	.619
2. Is there a tightness in your throat?	.595
3. Do you sweat?	.570
4. Do you tremble?	.534
5. Do you have shortness of breath?	.470
6. Are you worried about Pangols?	.360
7. Are you nervous?	.346

As a partial measure of acculturation to the urban environment, we attempted to construct a scale consisting of the following items from the social questionnaire: (1) Whether or not the respondent spoke French at the time of the study; (2) Whether or not the respondent read French language newspapers; (3) Whether or not the respondent favoured western style entertainment such as French language movies or discotheques over traditional activities and entertainment; and (4) Whether or not the respondent affected western dress when he or she returned to the Sine-Saloum for visits.

Among the males, the first three of these items formed a Guttman scale (Stouffer et al., 1950) with item 3 — favouring western entertainment — the highest point. The variables did not scale at all among the women. Upon inspecting the responses for each of these four items, we were struck by the fact that no more than one or two women read newspapers and relatively few spoke French. There were, however, many women who said they favoured western style entertainment, suggesting that there might be a group whose aspirations were out of step with the skills they possessed for participating in the European dominated aspect of city life. This stimulated a new research strategy. We constructed four different groups among the urban women as follows:

Group I — Women who preferred western entertainment to traditional, but who did not speak French.

Group II — Women who did not prefer western entertainment and did not speak French.

Group III — Women who did not prefer western entertainment but did speak French.

Group IV — Women who both preferred western entertainment and spoke French.

In 1975, we carried out follow-up unstructured interviews with men scoring

RESULTS

A. *Descriptive Health Data*

Blood pressure curves for both men and women, illustrated in Figure 2, are relatively flat. A multiple regression analysis utilizing age, age squared, and age cubed as predictors, systolic and diastolic blood pressure levels as dependent variables, demonstrated no significant associations. Furthermore, no significant difference was obtained between blood pressure levels for men and women or between rural and urban dwellers.

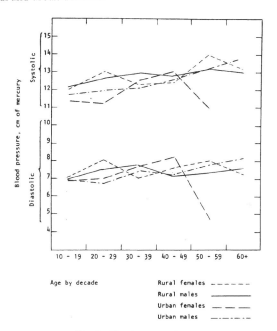

Fig. 2. Blood pressure by age.

B. *Descriptive Mental Health Data*

According to Figure 3 though 6, emotional distress levels for the rural group increase from the teenage years to age 20, thereafter remaining fairly stable until age 60. Sex differences emerge at age 60. Older men are at least as well off psychologically as younger men, perhaps a bit better. Women over 60 report more distress than men of the same age, and, on the Topical Depression and

Health Preoccupation scales, score higher than younger women. There are no stastically significant differences in scores of rural and urban samples at any age level or between sexes. In contrast with the rural group, it is the youngest urban migrants who exhibit the highest emotional distress score.

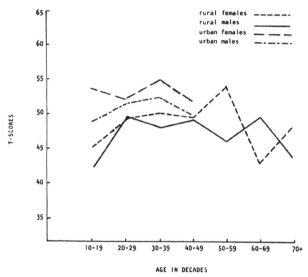

Fig. 3. Physiological anxiety scale scores by age and sex: rural sample.

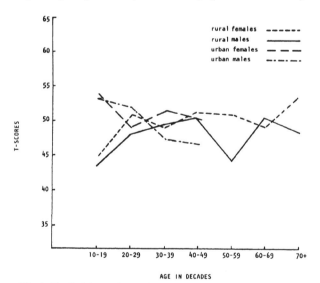

Fig. 4. Topical depression scale scores by age and sex: rural sample.

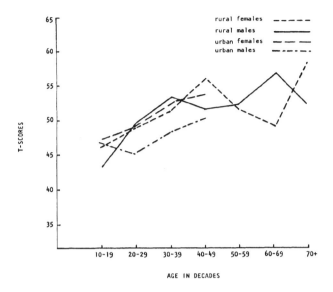

Fig. 5. Health preoccupation scale scores by age and sex: rural sample.

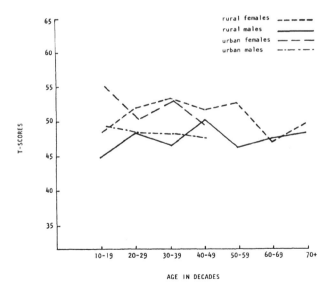

Fig. 6. Episodic anxiety scale scores by age and sex: rural sample.

C. *Mental Health and Associated Variables: The Rural Case*

Mean scores differed significantly by villages (Topical Depression, F statistic 1.90 with d.f. 10,225, p < .05; Health Preoccupation, F = 2.38 with d.f. 10,225, p < .01; Physiological Anxiety, F = 3.39 with d.f. 10,225, p < .001; Episodic Anxiety, F = 2.68 with d.f. 10,225, p < .001). Three villages almost consistently obtained the highest scores on each of the four psychological scales. With even greater consistency, two villages obtained the lowest scores on all the psychological variables. Village typologies for the three "worst" and two "best" villages with mean scores on each of the four psychological variables are presented in Table VII.

D. *Mental Health and Associated Variables: The Urban Case*

Correlations between psychological measures and acculturation scores among men are presented in Table VIII. In this table, we observe a weakly inverse relationship between acculturation and levels of psychological distress; the strongest association is with the variable, Health Preoccupation.

Table IX presents the blood pressure scores and Table X the psychological distress scores among the four different groups of women formed on the basis of a match between their levels of aspiration and the tools they possess for success in a strange environment. On each of these measures, Group I, those women who aspire to another mode of life but who lack the tools to succeed, achieve scores significantly higher than the other three groups.

E. *Urban Case Studies*

(In this section, names and some details have been altered in order to protect individual identities.)

Sagar, a Group IV woman — one who speaks and reads French and espouses western values — is married to Gadj, a government bureaucrat with a comfortable job and a guaranteed pension. They live in a suburban house furnished with sagging European sofas covered in flowered chintz. Sagar, who always dresses in the traditional bu-bu, occupies her day caring for her three young children, preparing cous-cous and other traditional foods, and visiting her Serer neighbours. Although she practices what some authors have called "role distancing" (Beiser *et al.*, 1976; Dohrenwend *et al.*, 1974) — disparaging her old-fashioned relatives who live in the bush — she visits them at least once a year.

Ann, another Group IV woman, teaches elementary school in a mixed European and Wolof neighbourhood. She looks very pretty in the western clothes she wears everywhere except when she goes home to the bush to visit her parents. When she does go back, she has to be prepared for the criticism her parents level at her for living with a European man. In the city, she sometimes cooks French dishes, sometimes a traditional cous-cous; usually, however, she leaves the cooking to her Wolof house-boy. Since she is fluent in French, Serer and Wolof,

TABLE VII
Village Types – 3 "Worst" and 2 "Best"

	I. VILLAGE FACTORS			II. PSYCHOLOGICAL MEASURES								
	Modern-ization	Exposure	Stability	Depression (m)	(s.d.)	Health Preoccupation (m)	(s.d.)	Physiological Anxiety (m)	(s.d.)	Episodic Anxiety (m)	(s.d.)
A. WORST											
(i) Village F (n=12)	Medium	High	Low	52.9	13.0	52.6	10.0	55.3	11.3[a]	56.4	13.7[a]
(ii) Village E (n=23)	Medium	High	High	52.7	10.3	56.3	9.1[a]	53.3	13.0[a]	53.6	11.1[a]
(iii) Village C (n=22)	High	Low	High	53.7	10.9[a]	56.2	10.7[a]	50.3	8.5[a]	52.7	8.6[a]
B. BEST											
(i) Village G (n=24)	Medium	Low	High	44.5	8.7[a]	45.5	9.3[a]	43.5	5.3	45.3	5.6[a]
(ii) Village J (n=21)	Low	High	Low	46.4	6.7	50.0	10.9	42.1	5.1[a]	44.0	4.9[a]

[a] "Best" and "Worst" Villages: mean differences significantly different for Alpha = 0.05 by Duncan's Multiple Range Test
(m = mean)
(s.d. = standard deviation)

TABLE VIII
Serer Urban Men: Acculturation and Mental Health

Correlations with level of Acculturation	1. Depression	2. Health Pre-occupation	3. Chronic Anxiety	4. Acute Anxiety
	(−.07)	(−.20)	(−.17)	(−.15)
p levels	p < .25	p < .01	p < .03	p < .05

TABLE IX
Serer Women in Dakar: Mean Blood Pressure Levels by Match Between Western Aspirations and Western Tools

Group	n	Mean Blood Systolic	Pressure Diastolic
I. Aspiration (+) Tools (−)	10	12.20[a]	7.40[b]
II. Aspiration (−) Tools (−)	37	11.84	7.19
III. Aspiration (−) Tools (+)	6	11.00	6.50
IV. Aspiration (+) Tools (+)	4	10.75	6.00

[a] Mean for Group I versus means for all others combined (P < 0.05) with 1-tailed test of probability.
[b] Mean for Group I versus all others combined (P < 0.20) with 1-tailed test of probability.

TABLE X
Serer Urban Women: Aspirations and Tools

Group	n	Depression mean scores	Health Pre-occupation mean scores	Chronic Anxiety mean scores	Acute Anxiety mean scores
I. Aspiration (+) Tools (−)	12	58.33[a]	53.2[b]	59.3[a]	63.0[a]
II. Aspiration (−) Tools (−)	41	52.0	46.1	50.5	44.7
III. Western Entertainment (−) Speak French (+)	7	44.5	41.5	47.9	47.8
IV. Western Entertainment (+) Speak French (+)	5	50.8	49.5	52.9	51.3

[a] p < .01
[b] p < .05

she frequently acts as an interpreter for friends or, in an official capacity, for one of the embassies.

Binta and Awa, members of Group I, value a culture in which they cannot hope to participate. Both are in a situation of double jeopardy because they have severed ties with the past. Binta is a Metis, product of a liaison between her mother and a Tobab (white man) who employed her as a maid. When Binta's mother returned to the bush, leaving her child with relatives in the city, it was not because she lacked maternal feelings. However, before she could hope to find a husband in Niakhar, her daughter Binta would have to be conveniently forgotten by everyone. Binta, never accepted by her relatives, taunted by other girls her age, dropped out of school at an early age and remains illiterate. She is now a prostitute. Awa became an outcast by marrying a man who became a tax collecter, the most despised and distrusted form of government official. Her Serer relatives and neighbours now shun her and her family. She in turn disparages them and their old-fashioned ways. However, being cut off from them and not being able to speak French in the cosmopolitan city, she often finds herself lonely.

Mahecor, 35 years old, works as a machinist in Dakar. At an early age, Mahecor began learning the history of the tribe from the village elders, who would sit every afternoon, at the foot of the great Boabab tree, telling their stories. Following custom, when his son reached age 6, Mahecor's father sent him to live in town with an uncle. Here the young boy attended school and learned to speak French. Afterwards, Mahecor's father who was now the chief of the family, sent his son to Dakar to look for work. A relative helped him to find a job as a mechanic's assistant. In the city, Mahecor joined a club called "Le Sine", an association of young Serer from Niakhar. Mahecor sent as much of his pay as possible back to his family in Niakhar and, on the average of once a month, went back home by bus. In 1971, after he had saved enough to pay the bridal price, he married a 15-year-old girl from a neighbouring village. Before any children were born, his wife came to live with him in Dakar. When she became pregnant, she went back to live in her father-in-law's compound. Mahecor, who interests himself in politics, speaks with some bitterness about the government of the still-young Republic. Although the President of the country is Serer, he comes from Joal which is in a more acculturated area than Niakhar. Under his leadership, the traditional Serer caste system and inherited system of authority is being officially undermined. As a nephew of the Bour, hereditary king of Niakhar, Mahecor would have been entitled to considerable power had official government action not stripped his uncle of all his authority. However, as an elected officer of his club, "Le Sine", Mahecor has become a leading force to preserve Serer traditions among his Niakhar peers in Dakar. This may not be all that unusual. According to my informants, most Serer who have been elected to the National Assembly come from the upper caste of Serer society — nobles and warriors. For Mahecor, and for most of his friends, the village is the only place to raise children: As Mahecor says, "One must really learn to speak the Serer language. First of all one must learn to understand the language because only in this way does a child learn where he comes from and who his parents are. I do not mean only his father and his mother. When one is a Serer, it is important to know his people." Some day, if he makes enough money, or when he becomes old enough to retire, he hopes to go home forever.

DISCUSSION

Serer who become urban migrants do not, as a group, display more health problems than those who remain in the villages. The survey data do, however, identify sub-groups at risk. Since these are cross sectional data, they are open to two different interpretations. The first interpretation assigns major causal weight to individual factors: it may be that persons with psychiatric problems are those most likely to adapt poorly to a new situation, by choosing to pursue valued goals which they are ill equipped to attain. The individual case studies suggest the reverse, that individuals become cut off from their traditional cultures, adopt unrealistic goals and then pay a price by developing symptoms of poor health.

Only longitudinal studies can confirm the pattern and elucidate the process. However, an expanding literature on migration and social change suggests that for most migrants, it is the interaction of social process and individual adaptive strategy which determines mental health outcome, rather than the reverse.

Figure 7, a model of the relationship between socio-cultural process, individual adaptation and mental health, summarizes some of the findings of this study as well as other relevant literature.

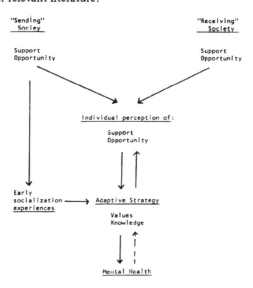

Fig. 7. Adaptation: social determinants and mental health outcome.

The pivotal variable in this model is adaptation, which comprises at least two dimensions — values and knowledge. Values are important in that they determine individual goals and also define for the individual what the appropriate means are for attaining valued goals. Knowledge, in the sense of instrumental skills, is important as well: if there is no congruence between valued goals and possession of skills necessary to attain these goals, frustration probably results.

Two macrosocial variables — the traditional culture of the sending society and the receiving society, constitute, according to this model, the major socio-cultural determinants of adaptation. Each of these systems potentially, or in fact, provides for the refugee emotional and instrumental support; opportunity to access the goals, material and otherwise, which the refugee values; knowledge about the means to access these goals and a set of values governing human behaviour from which he or she must choose.

The traditional culture also shapes early socialization experiences. Among these, the Serer tradition of sending young boys away from home to be educated by the maternal uncle — a pattern which Mahecor's father followed — is of great interest. Polgar (1960), in a study of American Indian boys, found that those who had lived away from home for a period during their formative years adapted better when they later effected a permanent departure from the reservation than those who had not had this previous experience.

In the Serer case, there is considerable interaction between the traditional culture and the receiving society. Urban migration, rather than signalling the disintegration of rural society, as some have suggested (see Assael, 1970, for example), has been adopted as a strategy to preserve traditional life in Niakhar. With insufficient fertile land to support an expanding population, families and sometimes even larger organizations within the villages, select young persons to become urban migrants. An understanding exists that this will be temporary. The young people are expected to continue to value traditional ways and to return to Niakhar when conditions permit. In the meantime, while working in Dakar, they sent most of their pay home and thus contribute to the village economy. Most Niakhar migrants in Dakar cannot, therefore, be thought of as having been split off from village culture. Instead, they exist almost as extensions of that culture in the urban setting. Dakar is relatively close to Niakhar, making it easy for migrants to return periodically in order to refresh their sense of cultural identity and to make it possible for the home village to reinforce the expected loyalty of the migrant. This pattern is not established immediately. A Serer migrant requires time to assimilate it, a factor which probably accounts for the pattern of association between emotional distress and mental health by age in the urban sample. Older urban migrants are probably people who have been in Dakar longer than younger. With time, they have, by and large, come to terms with this pattern. The association can also be partially explained by selection. Young people who do not adjust to the city are more likely to return to their villages; those remaining in the city are thus the most successful migrants.

The extension of Niakhar culture into Dakar probably accounts, in part, for the preservation of good mental health in the urban setting. Ben Tally, one of the Serer enclaves in Dakar, provides an example. An area of squat huts, small fly-infested restaurants, open market stalls and communal wells, Ben Tally houses a community of Niakhar migrants which reinforces valued behaviour such as pacifism and sharing. A voluntary organization, "Le Sine", to which many of the migrants belong, provides individuals with aid to understanding the new society, with companionship and with economic cooperation. The role of such voluntary organizations in providing support has as yet received insufficient attention in the literature on migration. (See, however, Little, 1965; Meillasoux, 1968; Murphy, 1977.) This type of support for individuals is probably only possible when a "critical mass" of individuals of like ethnic background accumulates (see also H. B. M. Murphy, 1977). The presence of this ethnic community makes viable a pattern such as that described by Group II Serer women, those who continue to value traditional ways over modern and who do not acquire the instrumental skills necessary to participate in modern life. Many Serer women in Dakar work, for a time, as maids, ultimately returning to the villages to marry and raise children. They may never learn French and may never need to if they choose not to participate in the larger society of Dakar. Like turtles living in protective shells, these women bring a closed psychocultural structure with them to Dakar. For many, the shell remains intact because they only stay a few years before going back to their villages. Some authors (Fried, 1964; Husain, 1956), however, have cautioned that this coping strategy is not a viable, long-term option: it can only be successful in the early stages of a country's industrialization. While the "turtle" style may be an adaptive pattern for some of the women, it is probably not available, even as a temporary option, for men. This is suggested by the inverse correlation between acculturation and mental health. Since most of the men must be prepared to spend a long time in Dakar, their chances of finding jobs and advancing will probably vary with their willingness and ability to modernize (see also Inkeles & Smith, 1974, 1976).

"Levels of hospitality", a phrase proposed by Aylesworth (1977) alludes to the receptivity of the receiving society towards new arrivals, the opportunities it presents to them, the access to required resources and the provision of formalized support. The level of hospitality which characterizes the receiving society is a determinant of adaptation, and of health outcome. In a study similar to our own, Scotch *et al.* demonstrated that urban Zulu suffered more psychological stress than Zulu who remained in the countryside (Gampel *et al.*, 1962; Scotch & Geiger, 1963; Scotch, 1963). Scotch attributes his results to apartheid, a policy which officially limits opportunity. Other authorities have identified migrants who are the "want-stimulated but achievement-frustrated" (Hughes & Hunter, 1970) as those at risk for developing mental health disorders (Barger, 1977; Kleiner & Parker, 1965; Leighton *et al.*, 1963; Marsella *et al.*, 1975; Murphy, 1977; WHO, 1960). Even though outside interests control a portion of the economy in Dakar, nationalization of industry under the rubric of "African socialism" is taking place under the leadership of a Serer president, and Serer are becoming increasingly prominent in political, academic and artistic circles. At a psychological level, the Zulu situation parallels the plight of migtant urban blacks in the United States. These three groups, living in white-dominated societies, are often denied access to the goals that the dominant culture defines as attractive. When people learn to accept goals but are then denied access to them, the response is likely to take the form of deviant behaviour, including mental illness (Barger, 1977; Dohrenwend & Dohrenwend, 1974; Jessor, 1968; Kleiner & Parker, 1965; Merton, 1957). For the Zulu, the U.S. migrant black, and the migrant reservation Indian, evidence exists that the relative powerlessness does accompany signs of emotional distress (Alfred, 1965; Boyce *et al.*, 1967; Gordon & Devine, 1966; Graves, 1973; Harburg *et al.*, 1970; Maill *et al.*, 1962; Stamler *et al.*, 1967). The Serer, with more options for behaviour open to them, do not, as a group, experience the same risk of illness.

Given the context of risk and opportunity provided by the receiving culture and by the traditional culture, individual destinies are determined further by what individuals come to define as valued goals and by the skills which they bring to their particular migrant situation.

For the Serer — men in particular — formal education, including the ability to speak and read French, becomes an important coping tool (see also Brody, 1973; Murphy, 1973). As suggested by the inverse correlation between acculturation and mental health, a man's chance for success in Dakar seems to depend on his willingness and on his ability to modernize. For women like Ann and Sagar, an ability to speak French means they can participate in a culture which attracts them. For Group III women, who are not interested in western culture, speaking French does no harm. Binta and Awa suffer, in part, because they are illiterate.

The "Turtles" as already noted, do not speak French and do not seem to suffer thereby; however, the attendant lack of flexibility may create a condition of health risk for these women at some point in the future.

Sagar and Gadj, the first generation of permanent urban residents, lived in Ben Tally when they first arrived; later they moved to Pikine, a new suburb. They now look back on some of their former neighbours — people such as Mahecor — as unambitious at best, perhaps even a little dimwitted. Nevertheless, even though both have largely replaced the value system with which they were raised with one in keeping with their new, modern way of life, they use their familiar culture for the support it offers. Sagar sees no one but other Serer in Pikine — women neighbours who think just as she does. Even though some of the ways of their families in Niakhar now embarass both, husband and wife still keep in touch with their home villages and visit occasionally. Sagar and Gadj are the "Assimilates".

In a study of first generation immigrants in the United States, Clark (1976) identified two typologies of adaptation. The first of these is a pattern in which individuals remain familiar with traditional values, consciously rejecting these values in favour of those espoused by the majority culture and assume "white face" — a pattern of behaviour that they believe will be looked on with favour by the valued reference group. This pattern, similar to the one described for Sagar and Gadj, conforms to the assimilation prototype in much of the literature on acculturation (Clark *et al.*, 1976; McFee, 1968).

Mahecor exemplifies a second pattern. He is capable of assuming "white face", behaviour expected of him in social situations when he comes in contact with Europeans or with Senegalese from different ethnic groups. He does, for example, joke about some aspects of Serer traditions when he is in white company. Mahecor also consciously rejects some traditions which he considers outmoded or destructive, for instance, the little known Serer practice of killing newborn twins. While accepting some values which seem "western" he does, however, remain intensely loyal to many Serer traditions — in particular, the subordination of the individual to the group. By moving with comfort between cultures, incorporating those elements most useful to them in the long-term, people such as Mahecor become truly bi-cultural. One author, impressed that the synthesis that people like Mahecor attain is a truly creative one, enabling them to live comfortably with two cultures — while most of us struggle to make our place within one — has called them the "150% men" (McFee, 1968).

Our epidemiological and case data thus identify at least three patterns which individuals choose to adapt to in new environments and which are compatible with good mental health. The "Turtle" style, which works for at least some of the women; the "Assimilative" style; and the "150% man".

Binta and Awa are adaptive and mental health casualties. Data from our study as well as others (Beiser & Collomb, 1981; De Vos & Miner, 1959; Fried, 1964; Inkeles & Smith, 1974, 1976; Kleiner & Parker, 1965; Leighton *et al.*, 1963) demonstrate a relationship between high aspirations, absence of tools and psychological distress. While the hypothesis that neurotic people aspire to things they cannot achieve is a plausible one, the case studies of Binta and Awa suggest that disorder is an outcome of their situations, rather than a cause. Not only are aspirations and opportunity out of synchrony, but neither woman can go back to her own culture.

It seems, therefore, on the basis of data gathered about urban migration that at least part of the reason the acculturative stress hypothesis often fails to be supported is that it is too simplistic. Another factor remains to be explored: it may be that the rural environment in Senegal is less benign than might be at first supposed. As Inkeles and Smith (1974; 1976) point out, the assumption that an urban environment is stressful may not be an error; the error comes in comparing that environment with a rural village and assuming the latter to be stress-free. Once again, our survey data suggest that the rural environment does in fact create situations of mental health risk. One can identify specific groups at increased risk as well as ecological factors at a village level which seem to jeopardize individuals.

For example, old women in Niakhar constitute a high risk group. So pronounced is this trend that it may account for the elevated scores of two of the villages — E and F — both of which number a disproportionately high percentage of elderly women among their inhabitants. (The large standard deviations in scores these "at risk" villages display on each of the psychological parameters indicate that not everyone in the village scores high, but rather that the mean scores are elevated by individuals or subgroups.) Is susceptibility to mental disorder a corollary of increasing age? If this were the case, one would have to account for the fact that older men display, if anything an improvement in mental health. Is there something, then in the structure or culture of the villages which creates stress for older women? While a Serer man's authority and stature increase as he ages, an elderly woman faces a different situation. As a young wife, she will have come to live in alien territory — usually, in her father-in-law's family counpound. It will have surprised no one — indeed it will have been expected — that she try to preserve the interest of her family of origin in this new environment. She will have insisted, for example, that her sons go to live with, and be educated by, her own oldest brother; she will have tried to promote a marriage between her daughters and her own male relatives so that the property which each member of the pair inherits will stay within her own lineage. When she is widowed, or if her husband should divorce her, she will expect to return to live with her family of origin and to be cared for by her eldest brother or his designate. At least this is what tradition dictates. The system has begun to break down under the pressure of overpopulation, sometimes leaving the old lady with a difficult choice. She will either try to return to her parental village and risk being rebuffed — or, at best, grudgingly accepted — or she will remain where she is and hope that people will be kind to her. In either situation, she will have become expendable. Social change has created a condition of risk for her by erasing a role which, in previous times, would have been available. One can predict that with improved health care making it possible for larger numbers of persons to live longer, the problem of the role-less elderly is not about to disappear.

Village C, one of the "worst" villages, displays almost the same profile as Village G, one of the "best": the former is high on Modernity, low on Exposure and high on Instability; the latter medium on Modernity, low on Exposure and high on Instability. Social dynamics could, however, hardly be more different. Village G provides a striking example of syncretism — the combining of old and new cultural elements in order to effect a new and unique synthesis. While the village is part of a successful cooperative, the management council is little more than a "front" for the traditional village authority: council executives are either family chiefs or younger relatives who act under the directives of their elders. The council has convinced the local authority to entrust them with the right to assign vacant lands. Thus, through a modern, seemingly new, governmental form, traditional practices continue and traditional values regarding authority are upheld. Contrast this with Village C where the government agent's appointment of young men of his choosing to the management council (including men of low caste) was followed by a confrontation between young and elders, between traditional authority and modern, egalitarian principles. Following the confrontation, many of the elders left the village. Although the people of Village C seem to be prospering economically, and although almost all who live there are Serer, ideology and tradition seem to be missing. This village, with its lack of clear cut patterns of leadership and followership, its cultural confusion, and evidence of wide-spread intra-group hostility, has undergone sociocultural disintegration and, as Leighton (1963) and Leighton (1963) have demonstrated, sociocultural disintegration is often associated with mental ill health. In this case, directed change which was too rapid and which undermined the traditional infrastructure seems to have caused this disintegration. Village G demonstrates that change need not invariably bring about disintegration. Why the difference? Why was Village G able to adapt by incorporating some elements and transforming others, meanwhile not jeopardizing the total sociocultural system? Delineating the adaptive processes in places like Village G, which apparently has been successful, and contrasting these with examples like Village C which has not done well, remains a fascinating question for further study.

Village J, which has not adopted the cooperative, but which has experienced high exposure, seems to be faring well. This village, one of the few in our sample to be situated near a major highway, has evolved into a prosperous market town. It is a large, ethnically heterogeneous place whose motto is: "Only good things happen". The Serer who live here have profited from the marketing skills the more worldly Wolof have taught them, meanwhile retaining a strong sense of Serer identity.

Several major points emerge from this study. Urban migrants experience social change. However, in the developing world, no one is immune from change, even those who remain in bush villages. For the most part, people adapt to change with less risk to their health than is frequently thought. Success in adaptation depends upon the support and opportunity provided by the traditional culture as well as by the new society. Success also depends upon individual attributes such as the type of value system an individual adopts and the skills which he brings into a situation of change. People who reject their past too quickly and adopt new values for which they may be ill equipped are people at risk for developing health and mental health deterioration. People who cling to the past, rejecting modernization, may succeed if the social structure in which they are embedded provides support and opportunity. It remains to be seen whether this is a viable long-term adaptive strategy. While change creates a condition of risk, it is also a condition of opportunity, a condition in which people are able to synthesize new identities. The last — which produces the 150% man — probably characterizes those who best adapt, who maximize the opportunity which change produces, while they master its risks. Their patterns seem close to that which Eric Erikson had in mind when he defined mental health as a condition of being "at home with one's family and with the future" (Erikson, in press).

NOTE

* Part of the research on which this article is based was done while the author was a Josiah Macy Sr. Foundation faculty scholar, 1974–75, and a member of the Harvard program in social psychiatry.

REFERENCES

Assael, M., German, G. A.
   1970 Changing society and mental health in Eastern Africa. Isr. Ann. Psychiatry 8, 1: 52–74.

Alfred, B. M.
   1965 Blood pressure changes among Navajo migrants to Denver, Colorado: A preliminary analysis. Navajo Urban Relocation Research Report, No. 9.

Aylesworth, L. S., Ossario, P. G. and Osaki, L. T.
   1977 Stress and mental health among Vietnamese in the United States. Preliminary findings of a mental health needs assessment among Vietnamese refugees in Colorado. Paper presented at the Health, Education and Welfare Conference on Mental Health Needs of Indochinese Refugees, Denver, Colorado, August.

Barger, W. K.
   1977 Culture change and psychosocial adjustment. American Ethnologist 4: 471–495.

Beiser, M. and Collomb, H.
   1981 Mastering change: Epidemiological and case studies in Senegal, West Africa. Am. J. Psychiatry 138(4): 455–459.

Beiser, M. Benfari, R. C., Collomb, H. et al.
   1976 Measuring psychoneurotic behavior in cross-cultural surveys. J. Nerv. Ment. Dis. 163, 1: 10–23.

Beiser, M., Collomb, H., Ravel, J. L. et al.
   1976 Systemic blood pressure studies among the Serer of Senegal. J. Chronic Dis. 6, 29: 371–380.

Berreman, G. D.
   1964 Aleut reference group alienation, mobility, and acculturation. American Anthropologist 66, 2: 231–250.

Boyce, E., Griffey, W. P., Nachman, M. et al.
   1967 An epidemiologic study of hypertension among racial groups of Charleston Country, South Carolina, in Stamler, J:, Stamler, R., and Pullman, T. N., (eds.): The Epidemiology of Hypertension. New York: Grune and Stratton.

Brody, E. B.
   1973 Lost Ones: Social Forces and Mental Illness in Radio de Janeiro. New York: International Universities Press.

Bruner, E. M.
   1976 Tradition and modernization in Batak society, in de Vos, G. A., (ed.): Responses to Change: Society Culture and Personality. New York: D. Van Nostrand.

Burgess, E. W.
   1955 Mental health in modern society, in Rose, A. M. (ed.): Mental Health and Mental Disorder. New York: Norton.

Carstairs, G. M.
   1973 Psychiatric problems of developing countries. Br. J. Psychiatry 123: 271–277.

Cawte, J.
   1972 Cruel, poor and brutal nations: the assessment of mental health in an Australian aboriginal community by short-stay psychiatric field team methods. Honolulu: The University Press of Hawaii.

Chance, N. A.
   1963 Notes on culture change and personality adjustment among the North Alaska Eskimos. Arctic 16, 4: 265–270.

Chance, N. A.
   1965 Acculturation, self-identification and personality adjustment. American Anthropologist 67: 372–392.

Clark M., Kaufman, S., Pierce, R. C.
  1976 Explorations of acculturation: toward a model of ethnic identity. Human Organization 35: 231–238.
Delpech, B.
  1967 Sociological approach to a Senegalese rural community: data and survey techniques. Psychopathologie Africaine 3, 3: 401–408.
De Vos, G., Miner, H.
  1959 Oasis and casbah – a study in acculturative stress, in Opler, M. K. (ed.): Culture and Mental Health. New York: Macmillan.
De Vos, G. A. (ed.)
  1976 Responses to Change: Society, Culture and Personality. New York: D. Van Nostrand.
Dewson, J.
  1964 Urbanization and mental health in a West African community, in Kiev Ari (ed.): Magic Faith and Healing: Studies in Primitive Psychiatry Today. London: Free Press of Glencoe.
Dohrenwend, B. P. Dohrenwend, B. S.
  1974 Social and cultural influences in psychopathology. Annu. Rev. Psychol. 25: 417–452.
Eisenstadt, S. N.
  1954 Studies in reference group behavior: I. Reference norms and the social structure. Human Relations 7: 191–216.
Erikson, E. H.
  In press Introductory remarks in Beiser, M. and Shore, J. H. (eds.): Flower of Two Soils: Native American Youth in Transition.
Fried, M.
  1964 Effects of social change on mental health. Am. J. Orthopsychiatry 34: 3–28.
Fried, M.
  1964 Transitional functions of working class communities: implication for forced relocation, in Kantor, M. (ed.): Mobility and Mental Health. Princeton: D. Van Nostrand.
Gamble, D. F.
  1967 The Wolof of Senegambia, together with notes on the Lebous and the Serer. London: International African Institute.
Gampel, B., Slome, C., Scotch, N. et al.
  1962 Urbanization and hypertension among Zulu adults. J. Chronic Dis. 15: 67–70.
Gordon, T., Devine, B.
  1966 Hypertension and hypertensive heart disease in adults. Vital and Health Statistics, Govt. Printing Office, Washington, D. C. (PHS Publication No. 1000).
Graves, T. D.
  1973 The Navajo urban migrant and his psychological situation. Ethos 1, 3: 321–342, Fall.
Harburg, E., Smedes, T., Strauch, P. et al.
  1970 Progress report: stress and heredity in Negro-White blood pressure differences. United States Public Health Service and Michigan Heart Association (HS 00 164–05).
Hughes, C. C., Hunter, J. M.
  1970 Disease and "development" in Africa. Soc. Sci. Med. 3: 443–493.
Husain, A. F. A.
  1956 Human and social impact of technological change in Pakistan, 1956, 2 Vols. Summarized in Textor, R. B. et al: Social Implications of Industrialization and Urbanization: Five studies of urban population of recent rural origin in cities of southern Asia. UNESCO Research Centre on the Social Implications of Industrialization: Southern Asia: Calcutta, India.

Inkeles, A., Smith, D. H.
- 1974 Becoming Modern: Individual Change in Six Developing Countries. Cambridge: Harvard University Press.

Inkeles, A., Smith, D. H.
- 1976 Personal adjustment and modernization, in de Vos, G. A. (ed.): Responses to Change in Society, Culture and Personality. New York: D. Van Nostrand.

Jessor, R.
- 1968 Society, Personality and Deviant Behavior. New York: Holt Rinehart.

Kish, L.
- 1965 Survey Sampling. New York: Wiley.

Kleiner, R. J., Parker, S.
- 1965 Goal striving and psychosomatic symptoms in a migrant and non-migrant population, in Kantor, M. B. (ed.): Mobility and Mental Health. New York: Charles C. Thomas.

Leighton, A. H., Lambo, T. A., Hughes, C. C. et al.
- 1963 Psychiatric disorder among the Yoruba. Ithica: Cornell University Press.

Leighton, D. C. Harding, J. S., Macklin, D. B., et al.
- 1963 The Character of Danger. Basic Books: New York.

Little, K.
- 1965 West African Urbanization: A Study of Voluntary Associations in Social Change. Cambridge: Cambridge University Press.

Marsella, A. J., Escudero, M., Brennan, J.
- 1975 Goal-striving discrepancy stress in urban Filipino men. II. Housing. Int. J. Soc. Psychiatry 21, 4: 282–291.

McFee, M.
- 1968 The 150% man, a product of Blackfoot acculturation. American Anthropologist 70: 1096–1103.

Meillasoux, C.
- 1968 Urbanization of an African Community. Voluntary Associations in Bamako. Seattle: University of Washington Press.

Merton, R.
- 1957 Social Theory and Social Structure. Glencoe, Ill.: The Free Press.

Miall, W. E., Kass, E. H., Ling, J. et al.
- 1962 Factors influencing arterial pressure in the general population in Jamaica. Brit. Med. J. 2: 497.

Murphy, J. M.
- 1973 Sociocultural change and psychiatric disorder among rural Yorubas in Nigeria. Ethos 1, 2: 239–262.

Murphy, H. B. M.
- 1977 Migration, culture and mental health. Psychol. Med. 7: 677–687.

Ness, R.
- 1977 Modernization and illness in a Newfoundland community. Medical Anthropology 1, 4: 25–53.

Ostfeld, A. M., D'Atri, D. A.
- 1977 Rapid sociocultural change and high blood pressure. Adv. Psychosom. Med. 9: 20–37.

Polgar, S.
- 1960 Biculturation of Mesquakie teenage boys. American Anthropologist 62: 217–235.

Rémy, M.
- 1974 Le Sénégal Aujourd'hui. Paris. Editions Jeune Afrique.

Reverdy, J. C.
- 1963 Une Société Rurale au Senegal. Aix-en-Provence, centre African des Sciences Humains Appliqués.

Senghor, L. S.
  1961 Nation et voie africaine du socialisme (Nation and African way to socialism), Editions Presence Africaine, Paris.
Scotch, N. A., Geiger, H. J.
  1963 An index of symptoms and disease in Zulu culture. Human Organization 22: 304–311.
Scotch, N. A.
  1963 Sociocultural factors in the epidemiology of Zulu hypertension. Amer. J. Public Health 53: 1205–1213.
Slotkin, J. S.
  1960 From Field to Factory: New Industrial Employees. Glencoe: Free Press.
Stamler, J., Berkson, D. M., Lindberg, H. A. et al.
  1967 Socioeconomic factors in the epidemiology of hypertensive disease, in Stamler, J., Stamler, R., and Pullman, T. N. (eds.): The Epidemiology of Hypertension. New York: Grune and Stratton.
Stouffer, S. A., Guttman, L., Suchman, E. A. et al.
  1950 Measurement and prediction. Studies in Social Psychology in World War II. Vol. IV., Chap. 1–9, Princeton: Princeton Univer. Press.
Tryon, R. C.
  1955 Identification of Social Areas by Cluster Analysis. Berkeley: University of California Press.
Tryon, R. C., Bailey, D. E.
  1970 Cluster Analysis. New York: McGraw-Hill.
Turner, R. H.
  1962 Role-taking: process versus conformity, in Rose, A. M. (ed.): Human Behavior and Social Processes, Boston: Houghton Mifflin.
United Nations
  1964 Planning For Balanced Social and Economic Development: Six Country Case Studies, New York, United Nations Publication.
World Health Organization
  1960 Health Aspects of Urbanization in Africa. WHO Chronicles, 14: 173–179.

K. Y. MAK, M.B., B.S., M.R.C.Psych., D.P.M. and
SYLVIA C. L. CHEN, M.B., B.S., M.R.C.Psych. (Hong Kong)

MENTAL HEALTH OF MAINLAND CHINESE IN HONG KONG

Hong Kong, the 'Pearl of the Orient', is a small territory of about 400 square miles. Of this area, just over one-fifth of the land is immediately usable. Yet, it has a population comparable to that of Norway, Guinea, Niger, or the Domincan Republic. Hence it is one of the most densely populated places in the world. This is shown in Table I.

Hong Kong's natural harbour and geographic position has made it a port of call on major shipping routes, and its geographic position and political stability have contributed to the development of communications by air. Moreover, the government has provided the right sort of environment to permit the interplay of market forces, thus making Hong Kong one of the most modern and busiest industrialized and commercialized centres in South-East Asian.

TABLE I
Population Density: land area (persons/km)

District	1961	1966	1971	1976
Hong Kong Island	13,303	13,637	12,809	25,400
Kowloon	38,979	47,505	42,860	
New Territories	384	397	468	554

More than 98% of the population in Hong Kong can be described as Chinese on the basis of language. The total estimated population at the end of 1976 was 4,477,600, the most recent figures available.

About 50% of the people is of Hong Kong birth, the rest being mostly immigrants coming mainly from the Kwangtung Province in China. The biggest influx of population was between the late 1940's and the early 1950's (i.e., during the civil war in China).

Among the immigrants who have entered Hong Kong are a group of Indonesian Chinese who, on their way back to Indonesia, failed to secure authority to enter there, and found themselves stranded in Hong Kong.

MAINLAND CHINESE IN HONG KONG

The inflow of immigrants from China during the late 40's and early 50's numbered over 1 1/2 million persons. Since then, there has been a continuous influx across the China-Hong Kong border. According to the Reports of the Director of Immigration (1975/76), the average number of persons legally entering Hong Kong is about 65 per day. The total annual number of such immigrants for the past few years were as shown in Table II:

TABLE II
Immigration From China

Year	No.
1972/73	24,540
1973/74	55,709
1974/75	32,057
1975/76	23,554

The figures for legal immigration, however, do not tell the whole story. In addition to this influx, there has also been a considerable number of illegal immigrants. While some of these persons have been repatriated to the Mainland, many others were allowed to remain.

A considerable number of those who have entered Hong Kong have been successfully resettled abroad, especially to North America.

MENTAL HEALTH SERVICE IN HONG KONG

Prior to 1949, patients suffering from mental illness were sent to a 'lunatic asylum' which provided only custodial care, with periodic transferral of patients to China. This practice was brought to an abrupt end by the founding of the People's Republic of China in 1949. The Hong Kong Government then took up the whole responsibility, and the Mental Health Service was subsequently set up and expanded. At present, the psychiatric facilities comprise the components listed in Table III.

The Mental Health Service also works in close co-operation with other government departments, particularly the Social Welfare Department and Special-Education Section of the Education Department. A number of voluntary agencies also take part in the rehabilitation of the mentally ill and in the promotion of better mental health in the community.

MENTAL HEALTH ASPECTS OF THE MAINLAND CHINESE

According to Morrison (1973), a number of variables may affect the incidence of mental illness among an immigrant population. These include:
    A.   Variables operating prior to migration —
        1. Personality of migrant
        2. Life experiences
        3. Cultural background
        4. Reason for leaving old environment
        5. Reason for moving to new location

TABLE III
Mental Health Service Facilities in Hong Kong

Mental Health Centres	Psychiatric Hospitals	Psychiatric Units	Psychiatric Clinics
(out-patients and day centre)	(in-patients)	(in-patients, out-patients and day centre)	(out-patients)
Hong Kong Psychiatric Centre (Headquarters of Mental Health Service (1971[1])	Castle Peak Hospital (1,921 beds) (1961[1]) Lai Chi Kok Hospital (300 beds) (1974[1])	Kowloon Hospital Psychiatric Unit (67 beds) (1971[1])	Queen Elizabeth Hosp. Psychiatric Clinic (1962[1])
Yaumatei Psychiatric Centre (1967[1])	[2] Siu Lam Psychiatric Centre (200 beds for	[3] Queen Mary Hosp. Psychiatric Unit (15 beds) (1971[1])	Tsuen Wan Psychiatric Clinic (1961[1])
Kwai Chung Psychiatric Centre (1977[1])	mental ill offenders) (1972[1]) [2] Siu Lam Subnormal Hospital (200 beds for the severely subnormal) (1972[1]) Kowloon Hospital Psycho-geriatric Unit (36 beds) (1977[1])	[4] United Christian Hospital Psych. Unit (28 beds) (1974[1]) [5] Princess Margaret Hospital Psychiatric Wing (1980[1])	Miscellaneous Sunday Psychiatric Clinics

1. Year of opening
2. The Mental Health Service Provides visiting psychiatrists to these two institutions
3. Run by the University Psychiatric Department
4. Run by a subsidized hospital.
5. Under construction.

    B.   Variables operating during migration — Stress of move
    C.   Variables operating after migration —
        1. Attitude of environment to migrant
        2. Homogeneity of immediate environment
        3. Fulfillment of expectations and aspirations
        4. Personality of migrant

For our Mainland Chinese, the following points are especially worth mentioning:

1. *Disenchantment on Arrival*: Many immigrants came with a hope of finding an Utopia in Hong Kong. However, sooner or later they become aware of problems of the new environment, and then look back with nostalgia to their own cultural norms (Brink & Saunders, 1976).

2. *Poverty and lack of family resources*: Unless they have close relatives who are willing to support them, the immigrants usually find themselves lonely and alienated. When compared to those who enjoy a rather extravagant life (as the standard of living can be quite high in Hong Kong), the immigrants consider themselves unduly poor.

3. *Housing problem and urbanization*: Owing to poverty and lack of supportive relatives, many immigrants have no recourse but to reside in the lowest standard of houses, e.g., in the resettlement estates (match-box like); or in the licensed areas. Some even have to live in huts or squatter areas. Most of these living places lack suitable space or public amenities. Moreover, as people are packed closely together, inter-personal conflicts can easily start off quarrels and disputes, and soon these generate a very high level of emotional strain. This fact was uncovered by a study (Lo, 1976) which showed, among other things, that the mental patient population in Hong Kong is over-represented in the resettlement estates and in low-cost housing areas (see Table IV).

TABLE IV
Types of Living Quarters and Mental Patient Population [a]

Type of Living Quarter	General Population in H.K. Island	H.K.P.C. Patients
	(1974) [a] (N = 222,940)	(1974) (N = 1,002)
Hut or squatter	20,716 (9.3%)	101 (10.1%)
Resettlement estates & low cost housing [b]	16,639 (7.5%)	166 (16.6%)
Housing Authority Society	17,174 (7.7%)	66 (6.6%)
Privately owned or rented [b]	163,022 (73.1%)	571 (57.0%)
Others	5,387 (2.4%)	98 (9.8%)

[a] Data available for 1974 only.
[b] Difference between the general population and the patient population is statistically significant. In these categories ($p < 0.01$).

4. *Job and employment*: While in China, the people are given work to do by the government but in Hong Kong, the immigrants must hunt for jobs themselves. Competition is extremely keen in this aspect, and in many cases, little job satisfaction is obtained. This puts an additional stress on the immigrants' mental state.

5. *Dialect and communication barrier*: Generally speaking, language barrier has been ranked as a major problem for immigrant populations to overcome. In the Hong Kong setting, it is rather the 'dialect barrier' which exists. People from different provinces of China speak different dialects while the Hong Kong-born Chinese speak mainly Cantonese.

With all of these factors acting together, one may expect to find quite a number of Mainland Chinese coming to the psychiatric centres for treatment. However, it is the impression of many psychiatrists in Hong Kong that the Chinese have a particular resistance to using psychiatric services. This may be so because: (1) there is still, among the Chinese, significant stigma attached to mental illness which deters people from attending; and (2) many families would bring their relatives with mental symptoms to private medical practitioners first, where they are symptomatically treated. It is only when patients deteriorate into graver conditions that there is a willingness to go to a psychiatric centre.

DISEASE PATTERN AMONG THE MAILAND CHINESE IN A PSYCHIATRIC UNIT

So far, there are very few studies on the problem of mental illness among the Mainland Chinese in Hong Kong. One study of 2,415 patients (1,205 males and 1,210 females) who attended the out-patient department of the Kowloon Hospital Psychiatric Unit during a seven months period from January 1st to July 31st, 1977, revealed 114 patients who were Chinese immigrants. These patients were found to have had a history of mental illness before arrival, or have experienced the onset of illness within 5 years of arrival to Hong Kong (see Table V).

TABLE V
Background of Patients Attending Psychiatric Unit

Category	No.	%
1. Immigrants from China, with onset of mental illness within 5 yrs. of arrival	52	45.6%
2. Immigrants from China, with onset of mental illness before arrival	48	42.1%
3. Immigrants from Macao	5	4.4%
4. Immigrants originally from Indonesia, but had returned to China	7	6.1%
5. Immigrants from other countries	2	1.8%

The data in Table V (Categories 1 and 2) show 100 cases of patients at the Psychiatric Unit who are immigrants from China; and of these, 52 cases experienced the onset of illness within 5 years after arrival to Hong Kong, and 48 other cases were known to have experienced the onset of illness before coming to Hong Kong. A further analysis is given of these 100 cases with regard to their diagnostic categories. These data are given in Table VI.

TABLE VI
Diagnostic Categories of Mainland Chinese Patients

Diagnosis	Onset of Illness After Arrival				Onset of Illness Before Arrival			
	Male	Female	Total	%	Male	Female	Total	%
1. Schizophrenia	18	10	28	53.8	18	8	26	54.2
2. Affective psychosis	1	2	3	5.8	1	3	4	8.3
3. Organic psychosis and dementia	1	0	1	1.9	1	1	2	4.2
4. Neurosis	7	11	18	34.6	2	2	4	8.3
5. Others (epilepsy and mental retardation	1	1	2	3.8	7	5	12	25.0
	28	24	52	100%	29	19	48	100%

In Table VI, a significant statistical difference is found between the patterns of illness exhibited by those with onset of illness after arrival to Hong Kong and those with onset of illness before coming ($p = 0.01$). Looking more closely at this Table, the following observations are of interest:

(1) There is a considerable number of patients with a diagnosis of schizophrenia in both groups of patients (over one-half in each case). Among the patients with onset of illness while in China, many admitted coming to Hong Kong for medical treatment. Hence, we may be seeing here a form of selective migration.

(2) This may also explain the high percentage of epileptics and mental retardates among the group of patients with onset of illness before coming to Hong Kong.

(3) There is quite a discrepancy between the percentages of neurotics in the two groups. The reason for this is not immediately clear. The effects of factors such as marital and family status, sex differences, occupation, education and place of accommodation need to be studied further. One impression we have is that a significant number of male patients who developed schizophrenia after arrival came to Hong Kong illegally.

Looking back to Table V, we find 7 patients who were born in Indonesia, but had returned to China during the 1960's. These Indonesian Chinese are now stranded in Hong Kong because they were allowed to leave China, but were not accepted by Indonesia. Of these 7 patients, 6 were diagnosed to be suffering from schizophrenia. This finding surely needs further investigation, but the sample here is too small. Perhaps the pooling together of cases from various centres can reveal a clearer picture.

CONCLUSION

A vast proportion of the population in Hong Kong, especially the older generation, are in fact immigrants from China. Many of them came between the late 1940's and early 1950's. Since then, there has been a continuous influx of immigrants into Hong Kong, either legally or illegally. The high density of living here, together with the rapid urbanization, the dialect barrier, and other stress factors, can create a high level of emotional strain among the migrants, which in turn is particularly deleterious to those whose mental status were already unstable while in China.

The Mental Health Service in Hong Kong serves the whole population, and a review of its service is presented in this paper together with a brief glance at the statistics of the Mainland Chinese attending a psychiatric out-patient clinic. These show that there is a significant difference in the patterns of mental illness between those who had their onset of illness while in China and those who developed their illness after arrival in Hong Kong. While there is evidence to suggest that the former group includes persons who come to Hong Kong expressly for medical treatment, the explanation for the different patterns of illness is not clear, and the need for further research into this phenomenon is certainly indicated.

The above presentation is based on the first exploratory study of the mental health of the immigrants from Mainland China attending the Kowloon Hospital Psychiatric Unit. We sincerely wish that this will act as a stimulus for further research. At this juncture, we would like to thank our Consultant Psychiatrist in-charge, Dr. W. H. Lo for his encouragement, and many of our colleagues for their advice.

REFERENCES

Brink, P. J. and Saunders, J. M.
    1976 Transcultural Nursing, A Book of Reading (ed. P. J. Brink), p. 126, New Jersey, Prentice-Hall Inc.
Cox, J. L.
    1977 Aspects of transcultural psychiatry. British Journal of Psychiatry 130: 211–221.
Department of Immigration
    1975–76 Annual Department Report.

Department of Immigration
 1977 Hong Kong Annual Report.
Lo, W. H.
 1976 Urbanization and psychiatric disorders – The Hong Kong scene, Acta Psychiat. Scand., 54; 174–183.
Morrison, S. D.
 1973 Intermediate variables in the association between migration and mental illness. The International Journal of Social Psychiatry 19: 60–65.

RICHARD C. NANN, D.S.W. and LILIAN TO, M.S.W.

EXPERIENCES OF CHINESE IMMIGRANTS IN CANADA: (A) BUILDING AN INDIGENOUS SUPPORT SYSTEM

INTRODUCTION

The importance of indigenous ethnic institutions as sources of social support for minority immigrants has been noted in several studies (Breton, 1964; Murphy, 1973; Nann and Stewart, 1975). For example, data gathered on refugees resettled after World War II in Great Britain, Australia, Canada, and Singapore consistently showed that where an immigrant group constituted a large proportion of the population, their relative rates of mental illness were lower than where they constituted a small percentage (Murphy, 1955). Studies of ethnic subsystems in North American society (Wirth, 1928; Gans, 1958) have indicated that ethnic institutions perform at least three general functions for their members:

(1) They provide a protective structure against hostility or rejection on the part of the larger society;

(2) They maintain objective and subjective elements of a cultural tradition; and

(3) They provide interest groups for the pursuit of particular political, economic, and cultural goals.

In addition to these general functions, ethnic support systems may also provide some very specialized services of a practical nature to meet the immediate needs of a newcomer. These may include such help as the securing of housing and employment, language translation and interpretation, advice and counselling, and connecting the immigrant with family members still in the home country.

There are, undoubtedly, countless occasions when the foregoing sorts of help are exchanged between members of the same ethnic group through a chance or informal contact. On the other hand, we have witnessed in recent years the emergence of formally organized ethnic social services in North America (Nann and Stewart, 1975). These newer forms of organization differ in one important aspect from indigenous structures which appeared at the time an ethnic community system first came into being. Whereas the latter have tended to be more concerned with helping members to maintain ties to their own ethnic institutions (Willmott, 1964), the newer forms of organization tend to be more concerned with helping members in their relations with, and adaptations to, social institutions in the larger main stream society.

In this paper, the experiences of an ethnic organization set up with the express purpose of assisting Chinese immigrants and Southeast Asian refugees to settle in Canada are examined. Located in the city of Vancouver, the name of this organization is The United Chinese Community Enrichment Services Society, better known locally by the acronym, SUCCESS. With the aid of a start-up grant of funds from the Canadian federal government in 1974, this organization has subsequently become an autonomous non-governmental agency, supported in the main by the local community.

IMMIGRATION AND REFUGEE SETTLEMENT

There are, today, nearly 100,000 persons of Chinese origin living in the province of British Columbia, with the majority residing in the city of Vancouver. This population constitutes the sixth largest ethnic group in the province, and is one of the largest minority groups in Vancouver. Historically, Chinese immigrants have been a part of Canadian society since their first migrating from California when gold was discovered in British Columbia. Another large group arrived during this same period comprising 15,000 labourers who were imported from China to help construct the western-most portion of the Canadian Pacific Railway. Anti-oriental legislation then effectively blocked further entry of Chinese immigrants into Canada until 1947, when close relatives were allowed to join family members already here. Following the removal of discriminatory parts of Canadian immigration laws in 1962, and with expanded immigration policies implemented in 1967, there has been a new influx of Chinese immigrants into the country over the past decade or so.

More recently, Canada has embarked on a program to receive 60,000 refugees from Southeast Asia. Among this group are many persons of Chinese origin who are being resettled in Vancouver.

Although the new Chinese immigrants and refugees may be internally differentiated by such factors as their most recent country of origin and their language and dialect, they share some common problems of resettlement. These may be broadly generalized into two categories:

(a) Problems related to migration and uprooting, usually involving major social, cultural, and economic change; and

(b) Problems related to a minority group status in Canada, with the consequence that prejudice and discrimination may be encountered in areas such as employment, education, and housing.

Resettlement problems are most acute for a large number of immigrants and refugees who do not speak English, many of whom also come from a lower socio-economic background. Their status is reflected in census data which show that the average income of Chinese families in British Columbia ($9,165 in 1971) is considerably below that of the general provincial average ($10,677), as is the average level of education attained by heads of Chinese households (6.5 years as against a provincial average of 7.5 years). Relative to other ethnic groups in British Columbia, the socio-economic status of the Chinese ranks near the bottom as indicated in Tables I and II.

TABLE I

Rank Ordering of Ethnic Groups in British Columbia Based on Socio-Economic Indices[a]

Education Scores: Ethnic Groups in Descending Order		Income Scores: Ethnic Groups in Descending Order		Occupation Scores Ethnic Groups in Descending Order	
Jewish	61.9	Jewish	61.7	Jewish	65.9
British	53.1	Scandinavian	52.3	British	52.8
Japanese	52.5	British	52.2	Scandinavian	48.9
Scandinavian	49.9	Netherlands	49.6	Ukrainian	48.0
Ukrainian	47.0	Polish	48.7	French	47.2
German	47.2	Japanese	48.6	Netherlands	46.8
Polish	46.7	Italian	48.5	German	46.0
Netherlands	46.5	Ukrainian	48.4	Polish	45.8
French	46.2	German	48.1	Chinese	45.5
Hungarian	45.9	French	47.1	Hungarian	44.6
Others	44.9	Hungarian	46.8	Others	43.9
Chinese	41.3	Others	45.9	Italian	43.0
Italian	40.6	Chinese	42.2	Japanese	40.5
Native Indian	30.3	Native Indian	26.6	Native Indian	33.4

[a] Source: Lilian To, *The Socio-Economic Status of Ethnic Minority Groups in British Columbia*, unpublished Master's thesis, University of British Columbia, 1979. For the methodology in compiling SES scores, please see Note 1 at the end of this paper.

TABLE II

Rank Ordering of Ethnic Groups in B.C. Based on Combined SES Scores[a]

SES Index: Ethnic Groups in Descending Order	
Jewish	63.2
British	52.7
Scandinavian	50.4
Ukrainian	48.0
Netherlands	47.6
Japanese	47.2
German	47.1
Polish	47.1
French	46.8
Hungarian	45.8
Others	44.9
Italian	44.0
Chinese	43.0
Native Indian	30.1

[a] For methodology in compiling combined scores, please see Note 1.

AN ETHNIC SUPPORT SYSTEM – PHILOSOPHY AND OBJECTIVES

Since its start in 1974, the SUCCESS organization has directed its attention primarily to problems encountered by non-English speaking Chinese immigrants and refugees. A service delivery model has evolved based on the following 3 assumptions:

(1) In a developed country like Canada, the well-being of families and individuals is dependent upon basic resources controlled by societal institutions in areas such as education, employment, health care, housing, and so on. The emergence of social problems can often be traced to a disconnection or a lack of fit between the needs of families and individuals on the one hand and the availability and accessibility of societal resources on the other. Such being the case, immigrants and refugees newly arrived in Canada are in a particularly vulnerable position. Thus, the services developed by SUCCESS are aimed at the special needs of immigrants and refugees who encounter difficulties in "connecting with" basic resources because of language and cultural barriers.

(2) When such problems occur, planned interventions may be required both at the level of the family or individual and at the level of social institutions. The former may need help in making more effective use of existing resources, the latter in making resources more available and accessible, particularly for persons who are not familiar with Canadian institutions.

(3) The provision of service to families and individuals is not, in and by itself, sufficient unless service users are helped to become more capable of helping themselves. Moreover, the sort of change which is required often necessitates a collective, mutual-helping effort. An important aspect of the SUCCESS approach, along with a case-by case service, is that of community development and the establishment of social networks which can act as mutual support systems and as vehicles for social action and social change.

PROGRAMS AND SERVICES

The SUCCESS organization is headed by an elected Board of 15 directors. A core of two paid employees provides staff support to a number of programs operated by volunteers, although these volunteers are often trained professionals who give freely of their time and skills. Persons who use the organization's services are also encouraged to participate in turn as volunteer workers in reciprocation for the help they themselves have received. Additional staff are periodically employed to undertake special projects of a time-limited nature as these are required. The organization's basic programs include the following:

(A) *Informal Drop-in Centre*: Operating out of a store-front facility strategically located in Vancouver's Chinese community, this drop-in service provides help to persons with problems requiring language interpretation, information and referral, and short-term crisis counselling. A monthly average of some 400 cases are seen, with the majority bringing problems related to finding work and establishing rights to unemployment benefits. Other prevalent problems concern difficulties related to immigration procedures, old age benefits, medical assistance plans, housing, registration for English language classes, and filing of income tax. In recent months, there has been a notable increase in the numbers seeking help for family relationship problems.

(B) *Adult Education*: The organization's educational services include a formal program of English language training with daily classes in the centre. Weekend workshops are scheduled throughout the year to provide opportunity for participants to share information about common difficulties experienced by new immigrants and refugees. These workshops also provide a forum wherein the participants can meet face-to-face with representatives of various community human service systems who are invited to attend. With the advent of an ethnic language radio and television system in Vancouver, the SUCCESS organization has also made full use of the mass media as vehicles for reaching new immigrants and refugees.

(C) *Social Networks and Group Programs*: A social network comprising over 1600 members is the main constituent body of the SUCCESS organization. This network provides a vehicle for collective action which is generally concerned with the improvement of public policies and programs for meeting the needs of immigrants and refugees. From this base, several age-specific mutual aid groups have also emerged which function as support systems for youth, for parents of school-aged children, and for senior citizens. Since its inception, the SUCCESS organization has engaged in a number of social action episodes. One involved the mobilization of Chinese community organizations across Canada to influence the federal government's policies on immigration. Locally, SUCCESS initiatives have helped to bring about a better coordination of English language training programs for all immigrants, and have provided leadership in pressing human service bureaucracies to employ bi-lingual workers who can speak English as well as a relevant ethnic language.

(D) *Research*: In spite of the lengthy experience with immigration and refugee migration to North America, large gaps remain in existing knowledge about the processes and effects of resettlement. Previous research has given considerable attention to the experiences of European immigrants while experiences of Asian immigrants to North America have received comparatively little. In recognizing these shortcomings, the SUCCESS organization has sponsored several formal research studies on subject matters relevant to the settlement of Chinese immigrants and refugees in Canada. These have included a study into the patterns of use of social services by Chinese community families (Nann and Stewart, 1975); a demographic study of Chinese community households (Goldberg); and a survey of government-sponsored Southeast Asian refugees settling in Vancouver (Yuen, 1979).

PROGRAM OUTCOMES AND LIMITATIONS

During its formative stages of development, the SUCCESS organization encountered many of the same issues faced by any neighbourhood-based social service centre in North America (O'Donnell and Sullivan, 1979). These include issues of function (specialized, or generalized); issues of structure (professional direction and administration, or citizen participation and control); and issues of staffing (professional service, or volunteer service). The way such issues were subsequently resolved has brought about some distinctive features to the SUCCESS organization. These features seem to be consonant with a new form of social service delivery emerging in North American which Kramer (1973) calls "alternative agencies". Such systems are indigenously organized and directed; they stress voluntarism and a movement away from bureaucracy and professionalism; and users of service are perceived as constituents who are also directly involved in policy-making and service delivery. This form of organization enables the system to deal with a wide range of problems encountered by immigrants and refugees, and while a requested service (e.g. financial aid) may not be directly provided, the system stands ready to connect a family or an individual to the appropriate source for help.

Due to the breadth of problems and concerns brought by the population it serves, the SUCCESS organization's drop-in centre has developed into a "first stop" for many immigrants and refugees seeking help. The large majority (70%) of these service users are not known to any other social agency in the city. Evidently, most of the Chinese immigrants in Canada are able to settle into their new environment with a minimal degree of help from Canadian social service organizations but there are others with long-standing problems who have not been reached. For example, an analysis of the cases served by the drop-in centre uncovered a group of families and individuals who have been in Canada for as long as 10 years, and who were still caught up in migration-related problems. For many new immigrants, and particularly refugees, the trauma of migration and uprooting must be dealt with before any real settlement can occur. Some come to Canada with personal resources and with their lives more or less intact so that their requirement of the SUCCESS agency's centre may only be a very brief service (need for specific information, help in language translation, or help in filling out a form). There are others, however, who need counselling treatment for more deep-seated problems. Fortunately, the drop-in centre is able to refer the more serious cases to a nearby neighbourhood mental health clinic which employs Chinese-speaking clinicians among its staff.*

---

* See companion paper by K. C. Li and Heather Luk.

Because the established social resource systems in a city like Vancouver are highly specialized, the drop-in centre's "gate-keeper" function serves to minimize the risk of a member "bouncing around" trying to find the appropriate source of help for a particular need. Moreover, because the user of the SUCCESS agency is a constituent who maintains a continuing relationship with the organization, there exists a feedback or accountability system, however informal, which can track the outcome of cases referred to other community sources of help. The users of the drop-in centre are primarily a low-income working class population. Those who are employed are in occupations such as farm labour, warehouse work, trucking, restaurant work, and work in the garment industry. Many of the jobs are seasonal. As a general observation, this population places great value on self-support and self-reliance. In the economic sphere, their greatest concern is with employment, or lack of employment opportunities. Because many are engaged in seasonal work, unemployment insurance benefits represent, for them, the most significant source of income support. But this resource is also controlled by one of the most highly bureaucratized institutions in Canada, with the consequence that a very large portion of the drop-in centre's efforts is devoted to helping persons establish their rights to unemployment benefits.

The role of "an honest broker" between the immigrant and an established bureaucracy, such as an unemployment insurance system, is not always an easy one to perform effectively. On the one hand, the go-between functionary can be easily co-opted by the bureaucracy or, perhaps worse, a large bureaucracy can often simply ignore the "noise" created by a local neighbourhood organization. Continuing intervention by the go-between may often lead to frustration or, at times, to a problem of overdependency on the part of an immigrant client. While one of the main objectives of the SUCCESS program is to connect immigrants and refugees with established social resource systems in the community, there is often the case where the needs of an immigrant population call for a service which does not exist, and therefore, must be created. The registration of Chinese immigrants wishing to become Canadian citizens offers a good case in point.

In 1977, when changes in Canadian legislation shortened the time of residence required for citizenship eligibility, many Chinese immigrants made known their desire to become a citizen of Canada. By special arrangement with federal government authorities, the SUCCESS drop-in centre was designated as a registration office and quickly became one of the busiest such centres in all of Canada. As a spin-off, the drop-in centre also established what came to be known as "Pre-Citizenship Classes" for the purpose of teaching the substantive information required for citizenship registration. (These classes also provided an excellent vehicle for helping immigrants learn the English language). With the assistance of professional educators from a local community college, SUCCESS staff members developed a special curriculum and text book which has subsequently been made available to organizations serving immigrant groups other than the Chinese.

From the SUCCESS experience, it is clear that an ethnic support system cannot, and should not, try to duplicate services and programs which already exist in the community at large. Rather, its role is to supplement and to complement, and to prod and to pressure, if necessary, existing resource systems to be more accessible and available.

In this regard, a large number of government bureaus have mandates which bring them into contact with an immigrant population. In Canada, they include: Employment-Immigration, Secretary of State, and the provincial Ministries of Health, Education, and Human Resources. As well, a host of local human service systems have, in recent years, found increasing numbers of immigrant families and children among the population they serve (e.g., public schools, local public health, and community mental health centres). The problem of a disarticulation and a general lack of coordination between, and among, the various governmental departments and human service agencies is well known. Gaps in services are often created by institutionalized boundaries established by the various social resource systems. These are problems endemic to the way social services have developed in Canada, and they involve such fundamental matters as constitutional authority, the traditional roles of private and government social service organizations, and a general lack of comprehensive planning in the social welfare field.

The dysfunctions created by our institutional arrangements obviously have important consequences for all Canadian citizens. For an immigrant population which has the added disadvantage of language and cultural barriers, the maze of government and non-government human resource departments and agencies becomes, for many, an almost insuperable system to negotiate and to use effectively. This, of course, was one of the chief reasons which gave rise to the establishment of an ethnic support system.

NOTE

[1] The SES scores (*The Socio-economic Status Scores*) which are presented in the Table represent a combination of the scores which an ethnic group in B.C. is assigned by using an averaging procedure which takes into account type of occupation, level of education, and current family income. The scores for the three items were developed on the basis of the 1971 Census data, and were assigned to each ethnic group in terms of its population distribution at each occupation level, educational level and level of family income computed from the 1971 Census Public Use Sample Tape data.

The methodology used in deriving the socio-economic measures was based on the U.S. Bureau of the Census Calculations issued in 1963. The scores assigned to the SES component items were derived as follows:

(a) The scores for education were obtained by computing a cumulative percentage distribution of the total B.C. population at each education level. The scores assigned to each level of education was the midpoint of the cumulative percentage interval for the category.

(b) The scores for family income were obtained in a similar manner.

(c) The scores for occupations were calculated according to the combined average levels of education and employment income for a given occupation based on the 1971 general tabulations for B.C. The score obtained as a consequence was an average score for that occupation. Using the number of workers in each occupation, a cumulative percentage distribution was obtained. The score for a given occupation was then determined by taking the midpoint of the cumulative percentage interval for that occupation.

(d) Each of the average education scores, family income scores and occupation scores were calculated for each ethnic group.

(e) An average of the combined education, income and occupation scores was then calculated for each ethnic group to obtain the SES index.

REFERENCES

Breton, Raymond
 1964 Institutional completeness of ethnic communities and the personal relations of immigrants'. American Journal of Sociology 70, September.
Gans, Herbert J.
 1958 The origin and growth of a Jewish community in the suburbs: A study of Park Forest Jews. In M. Sklare (ed.), The Jews: Social Patterns of an American Group. Glencoe: The Free Press.
Goldberg, Michael
 1975 Strathcona Community Needs. Vancouver: unpublished research monograph.
Government of Canada
 1971 Statistics Canada, 1971 Census.
Kramer, Ralph M.
 1973 Future of the voluntary service organization. Social Work, NASW, November.
Murphy, H. B. M.
 1955 Flight and Resettlement. Paris: United Nations Educational, Scientific, and Cultural Organization.
Murphy, H. B. M.
 1973 Migration and the major mental disorders. In Charles Zwingmann and Maria Pfister-Ammende (eds.) Uprooting and After. New York: Springer-Verlag.
Nann, Richard C. and Stewart, Penelope
 1975 Community Services and Ethnic Minority Clientele. Vancouver: unpublished research monograph.
O'Donnell, Edward J. and Sullivan, Marilyn M.
 1969 Service delivery and social action through the neighborhood center: A review of research. Welfare in Review, December.
Willmott, William E.
 1964 Chinese clan associations in Vancouver. Man, No. 49, March-April.
Wirth, Louis
 1928 The Ghetto. Chicago: U. of Chicago Press.
Yuen, Paul
 1979 A Sample Survey of Vietnamese Refugees Known to SUCCESS. Vancouver: unpublished.

K. C. LI, M.B., F.R.C.P.(C.) and HEATHER LUK, M.A.

EXPERIENCES OF CHINESE IMMIGRANTS IN CANADA: (B) MENTAL HEALTH SERVICES

This paper describes actual case examples from the Strathcona Community Care Team, a neighbourhood-based mental health agency, in its service to the Chinese in Vancouver over a 3-year period of October, 1973, to October, 1976. Before we proceed to the case material, some background information about the mental health service is in order.

The Strathcona Community Care Team is part of the Greater Vancouver Mental Health Service, established in 1973. It is funded by the Provincial Government, and administered by The Board of the Community Care Society of B.C. This Team, like ten other teams in Greater Vancouver, has a staff of approximately 15 persons, including two psychiatrists and all of the relevant health disciplines. A distinctive feature of The Strathcona Team is its availability of bilingual workers in English and Chinese, including the author psychiatrist.

The Strathcona area of Vancouver served by this Team comprises a multicultural population of about 40,000, with two-thirds being of Chinese descent. Until the establishment of this Team, there was no known public service agency in Vancouver with such a relatively favourable ratio of bilingual workers for one ethnic minority group. Since its establishment, it is fair to state that the Team is gradually gaining recognition for its contributions to the mental health and welfare of the Chinese ethnic group in Vancouver.

The favourable resources of our team include:

1. Availability of free service, so that patient income is not an important consideration.

2. The promptness of our service.

3. Comprehensiveness of a team approach.

4. Availability of comprehensive information of, and communication with, other agencies.

5. Close liaison to the Provincial Mental Hospital through the joint appointment of a psychiatrist in both settings.

SOME GENERAL SERVICE STATISTICS

In the three-year period from October, 1973 to October, 1976, there were 1259 active cases in the Strathcona Community Care Team. Of these, 190 cases (15 percent) were Chinese in origin. (At the end of the three-year period, the percentage of active cases of Chinese origin has risen to 28 percent).

The clients of Strathcona Community Care Team are generally residents of the Strathcona area of Vancouver, its catchment area. For the Chinese clients, however, only 50 percent (99 out of 190) are residents of Strathcona. Of the remaining cases, most live elsewhere in the city of Vancouver, while some 6 percent live in other parts of the province. No significant difference is found between the numbers of male and female Chinese cases served by the Team. Insofar as age is concerned, the adult group (aged 31 to 50) is slightly over-represented but there is a good spread of cases over the other age ranges (Under 18; 18 to 30; and over 50).

For the whole period of three years, 38 percent of the Chinese cases were diagnosed as psychotic. However, this figure changed dramatically at the end of the three years when some 67 percent of the still active Chinese cases were diagnosed as psychotic.

Over the three-year period, a total of 127 cases were terminated. Of these, approximately 60 percent were considered to have satisfactory results. A number of these cases were referred to other agencies for further assistance. These re-referrals usually involved assistance in matters such as housing, financial aid, training, and education and employment.

One notable statistic concerning our Chinese cases is the fact that 83 percent showed some degree of family involvement.

Of the 190 active Chinese cases during the defined period:

> 106 Cases or 55.8% required treatment under one year.
> 20 Cases or 10.5% required treatment under two years.
> 25 Cases or 13.2% required treatment over two years.

We currently have 63 active cases on record at the end of the period. The summary impression of our statistical data indicates that the Chinese service component of the Strathcona Community Care Team has exceeded its geographical boundary in a major way in order to extend mental health services to the Chinese clients; that about 60 percent of our clients received satisfactory service during this period; that the age group, 31 to 50, appears to be over-represented; that over half of our clients required treatment under one year; that the constitution of our clients by psychiatric category (psychotic versus non-psychotic) has changed over the three-year period; that the majority of our clients received family involvement and this is indicative of the relatively strong family ties among the Chinese; and finally, that there is no significant difference in the proportion of males and females in our Chinese clients.

With the foregoing as a general background, we will now examine some specific cases involving our Chinese clientele:

THE LONELY GRANDMA

Mrs Kong is a 65 year old widow grandma, who has been living with her adult son's family for over two years. After her immigration to Vancouver, she developed conflicts with her daughter-in-law. Mrs Kong did not feel she was well received. She was often excluded from social activities. Her views on child-rearing practice did not agree with those of her daughter-in-law. Mrs Kong believed that she deserved a better life, now that she had successfully brought up her only son through an arduous widowed life at her own effort. Conflicts in the family lasted for over on e year, with her son caught in between. Through the family counselling services of the Strathcona Community Care Team, Mrs Kong finally agreed to live an independent life in the Chinese United Church Dormitory, with assured periodic contacts with her son and grandchildren. Financially, she receives guaranteed income for senior citizens and does not have to negotiate for support from her son. Our latest information indicates that she has been quite comfortable, and has resolved her life expectations one year after her independent living.

The above is an example of conflict between generations which is so common in the Chinese family. It affects more often the grandma, since grandpas tend to die earlier. We have examples of similar conditions where grandmas do not qualify for guaranteed income from the government. They then leave home to work as homemakers or baby-sitters, and are quite unhappy about their fate. The Chinese orientation has been to rear their children to the best of their means, and to expect a return of treatment by the children when they become too old to work. To be neglected by one's own children at an old age is a major disillusionment for the aged, and a potent reason for clinical depression. Such behaviour by an adult towards the parent would be socially censured by others in the Chinese tradition.

THE CHALLENGING HOUSEWIFE

Mr and Mrs Mah are a couple in their late 20's, of junior high school education, who immigrated to Vancouver three years ago on the sponsorship of a sister. Since immigrating, the husband has worked in a printing shop while the wife works in the catering division of the same company. Besides work, Mrs Mah takes care of two children who are in primary school. Conflicts arose gradually because the wife felt that her husband does not participate well in the household duties, and enjoys himself in gambling and other social activities after work. Another complaint of the wife is insufficient time and affection displayed by husband towards the family. The husband, on the other hand, complains that his wife has become insubordinate since their immigration and has been too demanding in family decisions. The conflicts eventually led to a physical confrontation, after which the wife charged the husband for assault, and left home with her two children. Through court referral and family counselling of our office, the couple met three times and agreed on matters of future social activities, financial control, household duties and child-rearing practice. The couple subsequently reunited. The charge of common assault was postponed indefinitely by the family court.

This case illustrates the traditional attitude of a husband from a lower socioeconomic Chinese family, who believes himself to be head of the family, tends to monopolize family decisions, and to relate to children only with authority.

Wife hitting is quite common and acceptable among their peers up to recent years. With the change of environment, his wife has now fought back. This is aided by her economic independence through employment, her more assertive nature, and her acceptable educational background.

THE MISFIT IMMIGRANT

Mr Moon is a 38-year old university graduate from Taiwan, who has a wife and a three-year old daughter. He received military training before immigrating and completed his B.A. in Japan. He immigrated to Canada in 1970 on the nomination of his wife's sister. He tended to be sensitive and introverted even before his immigration. Because of language difficulty, Mr Moon was unable to obtain a job commensurate with his educational background. He completed a short course in English for New Canadians, and became engaged in a series of menial jobs, such as bellhop and janitor. He gradually became suspicious of people, developed ideas that he was followed and was the target of a communist conspiracy. He became unable to hold his job. Meanwhile, his wife was working and tending their daughter with the help of her sister's family. Mr Moon became more and more frustrated, and began to ventilate his anger at his wife through verbal and physical means. He alienated himself from his wife's relatives as well. He was eventually admitted to a mental institution on three separate occasions. Although he would control his anti-social behaviours while in hospital, his mental state deteriorated each time he was discharged. His suspicions and unhappy experiences in life and at work always recurred from imaginary and actual life experiences. Eventually, he was detained in the forensic psychiatric hospital after a very serious attack on his wife, nearly killing her. He was finally deported back to Taiwan as an alternative to staying indefinitely in the mental hospital. He was a jubilant man on arrival at Taiwan, as observed by his escorting psychiatrist.

This exemplifies the sad fate of a limited number of new immigrants who are not well adjusted emotionally and who tend to break down with paranoia from stress. The military background and the language handicap were prominent in contributing to problems in this case.

THE UNFORTUNATE MAIL ORDER BRIDE

Mrs Chan is a 22-year old housewife who was admitted to the university Health Science Centre Hospital in a state of depression and psychosis. She married her husband after a minimal acquaintance in Hong Kong. The husband is 10 years older and is a chef by trade. Her actual life experiences after arrival in Vancouver did not meet her expectations, as her husband appeared to have painted a better picture of himself before marriage. Mrs Chan became miserable, was unable to relate to her husband's relatives, and had to live in a two-bedroom rooming house in the Chinatown area. She could neither speak English nor go out during the day since her husband worked and preferred her to stay at home. He worried that she might get lost or get mixed up with "bad company". Life was lonely and impoverished for this young woman of junior education, who originally fantasized an affluent life in Canada. She was hospitalized in a depressed and disorientated state about five months after her immigration. However, after a very short period, she left the hospital without permission, so that her case was referred to our office. After much effort in contacting the husband who was quite defensive towards mental health workers, further psychiatric care was proposed; but it was only after a relapse of her psychosis, and her proposed divorce in the family court, that effective treatment took place. Through assistance of the family court worker, family therapy and individual treatment were rendered by our office. Eventually, Mrs Chan recovered from her psychosis, gave birth to a son and from our latest contact four weeks ago, was living quite happily with her husband.

This case illustrates a common example of the 'mail-ordered bride' where a woman marries her husband through correspondence, with minimal or no direct personal contact. Each side tries to hide personal defects which can no longer be concealed after marriage. This is a modified form of the old tradition, when marriage was conducted by family decision, with no direct contact of the marrying couple. Such a marriage naturally leads to all sorts of problems, even up to psychosis as in this case. We do have several other similar cases on record to suggest that this is not an uncommon occurrence. In some cases, such marriages are complicated by child abuse with tragic outcome.

THE INACCESSIBLE PARANOID MOTHER

Mrs Fox is a 46-year old housewife of primary education, mother of two adolescent children, and second wife of her aged husband who is 30 years older than herself. Her case received attention because of gross behavioural problems of her 15-year old daughter, and 11-year old son. On inquiry, it became known that Mrs Fox had gross paranoid ideas toward all public agencies, including the school, social workers, and any stranger. This was stated to be related to her previous unpleasant experiences with the Communist regime in China, before her immigration. Her husband is senile, given to alcoholic habits and has been the victim of hemeparesis for the past three years. The family of four lived in a shamefully disorganized home, and was coping on marginal financial existence. Daughter has been involved in extensive delinquent behaviour and truancy, while the son attended school for less than one-third of the term. Mrs Fox closed her door to most public agency workers, and was usually uncooperative to those who became privileged with a reception.

Through ardent and repeated approaches by the bilingual Chinese workers of the Strathcona Community Care Team, the son was gradually reintroduced to school, while the daughter was assisted in making some social adjustment. The overall family counselling, however, was rated to be unsatisfactory, as the husband was physically unable and socially ineffective in contributing, while Mrs Fox was too distrustful to form any meaningful relationship. Medication had been adamantly refused. The choice of management eventually pointed to either the continuation of a supportive role, or an enforced committal under the Mental Health Act. Because of the precarious condition of the husband and the absence of suicidal or external social disruption, it was decided that Mrs Fox should be left to live her marginal existence, although at marked expense to her children.

Poor educational and social background, together with pathological personality traits, work together in this sad family to prevent effective treatment.

THE HARD-TO-PLACE PSYCHOTIC BOY

Harry is a 10-year old boy in Grade four, who was admitted to the child psychiatry ward of The Vancouver General Hospital on October 30, 1975 after four months of bizarre behaviour. He was preoccupied with the presence of ghosts, was shouting and hitting his mother, and was unable to attend school. He is the youngest of five siblings from a labouring family, whose parents are in their fifties. Father works in a bakery while the mother works in a restaurant.

Because of their irregular working hours and marked age difference from Harry, the parents had not been too effective in their parenting. Mother tends to overprotect him. Harry's problem appeared to develop when his older brother left home after marriage, and his older sister left home for a vacation. With the temporary loss of his effective parental models, and an increased demand from a new class teacher, Harry decompensated into childhood psychosis. Intellectually, Harry had had problems in learning and speaking English as early as 1971. A repeated psychological test in 1973 indicated a performance I.Q. of 89 on the WISC, with no sign of organicity by the Bender Gestalt Test. After a one-month stay in the hospital with moderate response to medication, the decision had to be made to his further psychiatric care. Rather than send him to a long-term residential treatment centre with language and cultural gaps, it was arranged that he be followed up by the Strathcona Community Care Team.

Close liaison with the family and his school teachers was maintained since his discharge. Harry was transferred to the care of his older married brother and was allowed to resume school in his appropriate grade. He received regulated medication, and additional assistance in English skills from a special teacher. The school pressure was maintained and monitored regularly, while social support from his classmates and teachers was well maintained. The boy stayed in school and was doing well for three years until he reached the normal limit of junior school in Grade 7. Three episodic crises of various degree were quickly resolved by prompt attention of the Strathcona Team Workers and liaison with the school principal. Today, Harry has returned home to stay with his own parents, had developed at a physically normal pace and has been devoid of any noticeable abnormal signs or symptoms for nearly one year. He is now in a special class for students with learning problems. His case history has been most gratifying to his school, to his family and to his attending mental health workers.

CONCLUSIONS

The above case histories are examples of the work of the Strathcona Community Care Team. All of them involved an exorbitant amount of time and mental health manpower. They involved liaison with school, social agency, family meetings and often prompt intervention at critical times. They may be taken as advantages of a community mental health team in which facilities and working conditions are usually more favourable than those available from a private psychiatrist, or any private agency.

Our case histories illustrate several types of problems which are somewhat linked to the Chinese culture and the adjustment problems of immigration. To a certain degree, these may be found in other ethnic minority groups. Service by workers who are bilingual and bicultural appears to be more successful than that provided by workers with less empathy with a particular cultural group.

Our statistics demonstrate that Chinese in Vancouver certainly have their share of mental health problems, but they appear not to be over-represented in the community. The fact that the proportion of active cases of Chinese descent in the Strathcona Team rose from 15% to 28% in a period of three years raises certain possibilities. It may mean that the proportion of mental maladjustment among Vancouver Chinese is not as low as commonly held. It may also mean that the case finding effort of the Strathcona Team towards the Chinese clientele has been rewarded. Once a dependable service is established, increased utilization follows.

The fact that about 50% of our active cases are from districts outside the Strathcona boundary suggests that a similar service to the Chinese group in other districts appears to be in need, and that agency workers are accepting the value and contributions of bilingual workers towards the service of a particular ethnic minority. The expansion of this service either in the Strathcona Team, or the addition of similar service in other geographical areas, appears highly desirable. This would be a plausible mode for service to other ethnic groups as well. A related phenomenon is the interesting finding of Dr Richard Nann, Professor of Social Work, U.B.C. In reviewing attitudes towards public service, Dr Nann found that Chinese in Vancouver tended to use Chinatown (in the Strathcona area) as the centre of most of their service needs, in preference to agencies located in their residential districts (Nann and Stewart, 1975). This would speak in favour of the establishment of branches of most public services in the Strathcona area, if service to Chinese people is to be effectively rendered.

The proportion of psychotic versus non-psychotic clientele also warrants some discussion. Over the three-year period, about one-third of our Chinese clients belong to the psychotic category. However, the proportion rose significantly to two-thirds at the end of this period. Previous research by Dr T. Y. Lin and the Strathcona Team members (Lin *et al.*, 1978), pointed out that in comparison to clients of Anglo-Saxon origin, European origin or Native Indian, Chinese clients tended to seek help from mental health workers at a much later stage, when the condition is relatively more advanced.* Our current statistics, thus, may indicate that we are uncovering more cases that should receive assistance. Another factor is that over this same period, increased numbers of bilingual workers of Chinese origin are being hired by other public agencies; notably the Public Health Department and the regional office of the Ministry of Human Resources. The less-disturbed, or non-psychotic cases are therefore being cared for by other agencies, while our team is given mostly the severe cases — the psychotic. In terms of age groups, the 31 to 50 years' group is over-represented in our clients. One plausible explanation is the changing attitude of Chinese residents towards Canada. Until the recent decade, most Chinese inhabitants in North America belonged to the class of "sojourners" whose orientation was towards their homeland — China. No matter how hard they worked, or how long their stay, their ultimate goal was to be successful and to return home. This orientation has undergone drastic changes, related to socio-political changes both in China and in North America. The recent Chinese who immigrated after 1950 share much less of this view, and a higher percentage of them are accepting Canada as their home.

Finally, it is our belief that the Strathcona Community Care Team has provided a very substantial amount of mental health services to the Chinese population in Vancouver. It is our hope that our practical experiences may be offered as tangible models for service to other ethnic groups and, in turn, we will receive constructive comments for the betterment of our current practices.

ACKNOWLEDGEMENT

The authors wish to acknowledge the efforts of their fellow team members, namely Mrs Mei-Chen Lin, Raymond Chan, and Andrew Mark, whose combined efforts made up the service and statistics of this report; and David Yeung who has contributed significant effort in the data collection. Also, our thanks to the Strathcona Community Care Team for their co-operation and consent in releasing the team information.

REFERENCES

Lee, Rose Hum
    1950 Chinese in North America. University of Hong Kong.
Lin, Tsung-yi et al.
    1978 Ethnicity and pathways of patients seeking treatment, Culture, Medicine and Psychiatry 3: 13.

---

* See companion paper by Mei-chen Lin.

Nann, Richard C. and Stewart, P.
 1975 Community Service and Minority Clientele: A Study Pattern of Social Services Delivery and Variations in Service and by Chinese in Vancouver, unpublished research monograph.

MEI-CHEN LIN

EXPERIENCES OF CHINESE IMMIGRANTS IN CANADA: (C) PATTERNS OF HELP-SEEKING AND SOCIO-CULTURAL DETERMINANTS

INTRODUCTION

In a recent study in Vancouver, Lin *et al.* (1978) found that the patterns of help-seeking of psychiatric patients differed significantly among four cultural groups investigated. The groups comprised Anglo-Saxon Canadians, Chinese Canadians, Mid-European immigrants, and Native Indians. The differential patterns of help-seeking would seem to have important implication for planning and implementing mental health services relevant to the culture and socio-economic reality of each group.

This paper will be concerned only with the Chinese group. We shall, first, describe the characteristic ways in which psychiatric problems were recognized and managed by the families. Secondly, we shall attempt to explain the socio-cultural significance of the peculiar pattern of management of mental illness in the Chinese families and Chinese community. Thirdly, we shall discuss its implications for delivering mental health services to the Chinese.

THREE TYPES OF HELP-SEEKING

The study referred to at the start of this paper involved a total of 77 patients served by a neighbourhood-based community mental health team.* These patients had the following general characteristics: (1) a fairly even distribution among all adult age groups, (2) few currently married and fewer living with spouses, (3) mostly unemployed; occupations listed as unskilled, and (4) approximately half received previous inpatient and outpatient care. The study uncovered three distinct types of help-seeking patterns among the four cultural groups represented by the patients. For the sake of easy reference, we shall refer to these as Type A, B, and C. They represent the following respective profiles:

Type A is characterized by early, intensive, and prolonged efforts by the family itself to cope with psychiatric or non-criminal anti-social problems of the patient. Very rarely are alcoholism, drug abuse, or suicides reported. The family's management of problems ranges from advice, moral exhortation, dietetic, herb and faith healing, to physical isolation or physical constraints. Later, certain community leaders (e.g., teachers, elders, and other members of an extended kinship group) are brought in for consultation in assist the family. Then lastly, family

---
* See companion paper by K. C. Li and Heather Luk.

doctors are called to see the patient. External agencies of any kind — social, psychological, marital, or legal — are rarely involved. Eventually, the patient is referred to a mental hospital. Upon subsequent discharge to the family, the attempts at intra-familial coping resume until the limit of family tolerance is reached, or available resources exhausted. Then, the patient is again sent to a mental hospital. The above cycle of intra-familial coping and hospitalization repeats itself time and again until the patient is ultimately rejected by the family to become the responsibility of a public institution or aftercare service within the community.

Type B is characterized by early referral to mental health or to social agencies, counselling, and legal services with minimal efforts at intra-familial coping with the patient's problems. Often, such referral is made by the patient himself. The most frequently reported problems are alcohol and drug abuse, psychosmatic ailments, and marital conflicts. Referral to psychiatric hospitals takes place after multiple attempts to enlist social or mental health ambulatory services.

Type C patients have few, if any, family interventions at any point in the pathway. When problems arise, usually a non-family person (e.g., a friend or landlady) alerts a social, medical, or legal agency for assistance. The most commonly reported problems are suicidal attempts, alcoholism, drugs, existential and social difficulties, or conflicts with the law. As a rule, the patient is handled briefly by one agency at a time, and then referred to another agency, and then another. This process of "passing the buck" often involves police, legal agencies and correctional institutions.

As noted in Table I, of the 77 patients included in the study, 20 belonged to Type A; 34 to Type B; and 10 to Type C. The remaining 13 did not appear to belong to any one type, most having a mixture of Type A and Type B characteristic features. They are aggregated as a fourth group. Nineteen out of 24 Chinese (79%) belonged to Type A; 18 out of 24 Anglo-Saxon Canadian (75%) belonged to Type B; 6 out of 9 Native Indians (67%) belonged to Type C; and 65% of the European immigrants to Type B. The association of ethnicity with patterns of help-seeking is most striking and found to have a strong statistical significance. (Table I).

Ethnicity and length of time in Canada were also statistically significant in differentiating patients in the various types of help-seeking patterns. Type A, mostly Chinese patients, showed a tendency of being the most recent arrivals in Canada, with an average residence of ten years. Type C, Native Indians, were understandably the longest residents in Canada. Type B, Anglo-Saxon and Middle-European, were intermediate with averages of almost 20 years residence in Canda. The data in Table II present a summary of episodes in each type of Help-seeking pattern, listed according to type of problem, person recognizing problem, and type of intervention. It is notable that here, too, the differences among the various help-seeking patterns are statistically significant.

TABLE I

Patients in each type of help-seeking pattern by: I. Ethnicity and II. Time in Canada

I. Ethnicity		Type of help-seeking pattern			
		A	B	C	(D)
		(Number of patients)			
Chinese	24	19	0	1	4
Anglo-Saxon	24	1	8	2	3
Middle-European	20	0	13	1	6
Native Indian	9	0	3	6	0
Total	77	20	34	10	13
$\chi^2 = 82.67$	df = 9	p = 0.00005			

II. Time in Canada

means [a]		3.8	1.88	1.10	2.59
F ratio = 9.90 (between groups)		df = 3	p = < 0.0005		

[a] 1 = born in Canada
2 = 20 years
3 = 10–19 years
4 = 5–9 years
5 = 2–4 years
6 = 1 year

CONCEPT OF MENTAL ILLNESS AND ITS SOCIAL STIGMA

The traditional Chinese view on mental illness seems to be still prevalent and dominant among those transplanted and living among Canadians in Canada. The fact that almost all the cases reported psychotic behaviour or irrational anti-social behaviour at the onset conforms to the classic, commonly held concept of "Feng-tsu" (the lunatic). The long delay in asking for psychiatric help, sometimes up to 20 to 25 years, can be in part attributed to the family's genuine concern to the well-being of its sick members. Stories of sacrifices which some families make for a sick member in order to cure illness are legendary (Berk et al., 1973). It cannot, however, be overlooked that the extreme reluctance of the family to expose the patient, or to admit the presence of the mentally ill in the family, to outsiders plays an important role in keeping the patient unduly long from available treatment. The social stigma and shame attached to mental illness in China is indeed widespread, severe, and complex. (Chen, 1976; Lin, et al., 1978). It is the combination of the above factors which confines a psychiatric patient inside the Chinese family for as long as possible. (Berk et al., 1973; Lin and Lin, 1978; Sue and McKinney, 1975).

TABLE II
Sums of episodes in each type of help-seeking pattern by: I. Type of problem,
II. Person recognizing the problem; III. Type of intervention.

		Type of help-seeking pattern Sums of episodes (observed) (expected)			
		A	B	C	(D)
I.	Type of problem				
	psychotic psychiatric	21 (.17)	30 (0.9)	5 (0.5)	9 (1.0)
	violent criminal	12 (0.8)	44 (1.1)	11 (1.0)	9 (0.8)
	antisocial non-criminal	9 (1.4)	18 (1.0)	4 (0.8)	4 (0.8)
	alcohol or drugs	0 (0)	19 (1.5)	4 (1.2)	1 (0.3)
	non-psychotic psychiatric	20 (1.2)	45 (1.0)	13 (1.0)	13 (0.0)
	psychophysiological	6 (1.0)	19 (1.2)	4 (0.9)	2 (0.5)
	suicidal	3 (0.6)	11 (0.8)	8 (2.1)	4 (1.1)
	social	6 (0.6)	22 (0.8)	13 (1.7)	11 (1.5)
	aftercare	5 (0.9)	15 (1.0)	1 (0.2)	9 (2.1)
	Total*	82	223	64	62
	χ^2 = 43.91	df = 24	p = 0.008		
II.	Person recognizing problem				
	self	5 (0.8)	20 (1.3)	3 (0.7)	2 (0.4)
	parents	20 (2.5)	7 (0.4)	3 (0.6)	9 (1.6)
	spouse	14 (2.4)	8 (0.6)	1 (0.3)	5 (1.2)
	mental health professional	33 (0.9)	97 (1.1)	16 (0.7)	29 (1.1)
	medical professional	14 (1.2)	26 (0.9)	9 (1.1)	9 (1.1)
	social services	11 (0.6)	40 (0.9)	23 (1.9)	12 (1.0)
	legal	0 (0)	37 (1.4)	11 (1.5)	3 (0.4)
	Total*	98	235	66	69
	χ^2 = 86.38	df = 18	p = 0.00001		
III.	Type of intervention				
	family	21 (2.4)	10 (0.5)	3 (0.5)	6 (1.0)
	psychiatric outpatient	18 (1.1)	42 (1.0)	7 (0.6)	18 (1.4)
	psychiatric inpatient	18 (0.8)	54 (1.1)	11 (0.8)	15 (1.0)
	medical	21 (1.3)	32 (0.9)	9 (0.9)	11 (1.0)
	social services	14 (0.8)	57 (1.4)	19 (1.6)	14 (1.1)
	legal	2 (0.2)	35 (1.4)	11 (1.5)	4 (0.5)
	Total*	94	230	60	68
	χ^2 = 52.28	df = 15	p = 0.00001		

* Note that totals differ as a result of unknown information for some episodes.

The Chinese view on the etiology of mental illness is complex and underlies their attitude and methods of handling the mentally sick. It has many components to it — moralistic, religious, cosmic, physiological, psychological, social and hereditary. The weight of each component varies from one individual to another, and even in one person, it may vary with time and under different circumstances. A moralistic view emphasizes two aspects of "misconduct" as causes for mental illness; firstly, deviation from socially prescribed or acceptable behaviour and secondly, one's neglect of paying due respect to a dead ancestor. In either case, mental illness is regarded as a punishment for violation of two of the most important moral codes in Chinese life — Confucian moral conduct and fillial piety.

Punitive implication is present also in the cosmic or mystic etiology of mental illness. It is regarded as the wrath of certain gods or deceased ancestors whom the patient or his family incurred in this life or in his previous life, as many Chinese believe in reincarnation. It is, therefore, understandable that shame and/or guilt is pervasive in Chinese families in the presence of mental illness. The physiological view consists basically of an imbalance of Yin and Yang. According to Nei-ching, the classic of Internal Medicine by Yellow Emperor, mental illness is caused by five harmful emanations affecting Yin and Yang. These five disturbances are numbness (痺), wildness (狂), insanity (顛), disturbance of speech (瘖), and anger (怒) (Ilza, 1972). Excess or shortage of such physiological functions as breathing, eating, bowel movement, sexual activity (including masturbation), physical exercise, or exhaustion are believed to upset the Yin-Yang balance, leading to mental illness. Excessive sex or abstinence is believed to be most harmful. Climatic changes also affect the above physiological functions, especially the sexual functions, in causing harmful effects on the balance of Yin and Yang. For example, manic excitement is often called "peach blossom insanity" as it is believed to occur commonly in the spring among the young with hypersexual manifestations. In Chinese, peach blossoms symbolize sex and youth as well as the spring season. As a modern addition, hormones and vitamins are included in the above list to cause imbalance of Yin and Yang. Dysfunction of the brain or the central nervous system is also regarded by the Chinese as a source of disturbance to the mind and the behaviour of an individual. These physiological or medical causations are almost always sought by the patient's family, and remedies such as special diet, including eating the brain or kidneys of animals and herbs, are used quite extensively. Often, traditional herb doctors or elders of the extended family are called upon for advice in suggesting and choosing the most appropriate remedy. Such "medical" treatment seems to offer a high degree of psychological relief to the family from their shame and/or guilt over the patient's mental illness.

The Chinese view on the etiological importance of psycho-social factors is comparable to the Westerner's. Failure in love affairs, loss of loved ones, financial disaster, etc., are readily regarded as responsible for a patient's mental illness by the family. To the Chinese, however, the breakdown of the family relationship seems to be given much more weight as a psychogenic factor than in other cultures (Fong, 1973).

Hereditary factors act upon an individual in two ways for the Chinese. One is the notion of biological genetic transmission of psychiatric illness. The other is the belief that the patient inherits the "disturbance" by virtue of parental or ancestral "misconduct" which acts as a "seed" for the patient's developing behaviour problems later on.

THE FAMILY'S RESPONSE AND INTERVENTION: LOVE, DENIAL AND REJECTION

The initial puzzlement and concern of the family over the gradual or sudden change of behaviour of an individual usually leads to typical mixed responses. Most commonly observed are attempts at correcting the behaviour by reasoning or exhortation on the one hand, and making light of the signnificance of such behaviour on the other. At the same time, family members do make every effort to conceal it from outsiders while discussions take place within the family over the cause of the abnormal behaviour, going over every possible etiological factor. Pragmatism characteristic of Chinese approach to problem solving, prevails in the ensuing process. Whoever succeeds in convincing the other members of the family of his/her view gets his or her way in trying out the proposed remedies. It should be noted that the person's hierarchical position in the family, including age, is a dominant factor in the decision-making process.

The view of the head of the family, grandparents or parents, usually takes precedence over the others. For example, if the grandfather holds the view of physiological or dietary causation, then herb medicine or a dietary regime may be tried first. Failing to achieve the expected effects, then the grandmother's view, say a cosmic religious approach, will be adopted. Certain religious ceremonies will be performed, and the offering of food and burning of silver or gold money will be made to ease the wrath of deceased ancestors or roaming ghosts. Following this, the father's proposal to investigate the patient's history may be given consideration, and the patient's siblings or friends get called in to provide information on the patient's life or love affairs. In this manner, one after the other possible causative factor is explored, and proposed remedies are tried.

Often, the same cycle repeats itself until the tolerance and resources of the family are exhausted. Usually at this moment, the medical theory comes to dominate and a physician, and later through the physician, a psychiatrist, is called. Failing in obtaining improvement, the patient is eventually sent to an institution. Repetition of the cycle of hospitalization and home care usually ends up in the eventual rejection of the patient by the family. The enormous effort put in by the family to manage psychiatric problems at home, and the pragmatic approaches in experimenting with one treatment modality after the other, definitely prolongs the home care of the mental patient for periods ranging from several to 25 years, (Lin and Lin, 1978). A patient recently referred for mental health treatment provides a dramatic illustration:

When a shabby downtown hotel was closed, a 32-year-old Chinese man, an occupant of a room for 12 years, came to the attention of a social agency in charge of rehousing the residents. The man was immediately recognized as having florid schizophrenic symptoms of hallucinations, delusions and autism, and was referred to mental health treatment. No one in the hotel, not even the proprietor, had known anything about the condition of the man for over 12 years, although his family had brought three daily meals regularly to this man, and he seldom came out of his room for all of these years. During the interview, his family, who live in an apartment, wished they could have had a larger house to take care of "the boy". The social stigma attached to mental illness with the strong shame and guilt of the family underlies this whole process, (Sue and Kitano, 1973).

"THEY" AND "WE"

The heavy reliance on intrafamilial resources of the Chinese is strongly reinforced by their cultural isolation and social distance as a minority group in a Western society. Language barrier and the effects of longstanding discrimination which denied them access to available social resources are all too evident (Sue and McKinney, 1975). Many social agencies — governmental or non-governmental — are not only foreign to the Chinese; they are regarded as representing the all powerful "Big Brother". The Chinese look upon them with awe and sometimes fear, and consider it best to have nothing to do with them unless it is absolutely unavoidable. Even then, they usually get someone they can trust as an intermediate go-between (plus interpreter) to be present. The distinction between "they" and "we" runs through every social interaction of the Chinese as individuals, as a family, and as a cultural group.

The roots for the distrust or distant attitude to "outsiders" goes much deeper and further in Chinese history. For many thousands of years, the trust and sense of security rarely went beyond the family circle, which is usually an extended one and often included those related by marriage or childhood friends of the parents. Only these people, being part of "us", are trusted and included in the formal or informal council of family dealing with matters of importance. Finance, education, marriage, health, or any family discord affecting any of the individuals, are the concern of this inner circle of the close-knit family. Leaking of information or exposure of family discord to outsiders are regarded as "loss of face" and a serious disgrace to the family. The sphere of privacy has three concentric circles extending from the individual, to the immediate family, and then to the wider extended family circle. Language plays an important role in differentiating between "them" and "us". The people who speak their tongue or dialect are almost instantly recognized as one of "us", and those who do not are regarded as outsiders with an instantaneous response of suspect accorded to a foreigner.

The Chinese immigrants carried this family centralism with them to foreign shores and drew from it their security and sense of identity. The social discrimination and language barrier reinforced their attitude, and drove from to withdraw further into their family shell, almost to the extent of "cultural autism", especially amongst the first generation immigrants. Although the successive generations gradually adopted some of the Western life style, including Western attitudes to family affairs and the concept of individualism (Fong, 1973; Mead, 1970), there is no denying that the traditional Chinese way still prevails (Ho, 1976).

Emphasis on shared responsibility and loyalty to the well-being of family members makes Chinese less interested in, and sometimes neglectful of, the well-being of outsiders. The Western concept of community or citizenship responsibility makes sense to them only when translated into family terms. The fact that few overseas Chinese concern themselves with politics or engage in human services speaks for this attitude. This lack of social or political interest in the community further lessens the chances of their utilizing or developing extrafamilial social resources.

SERVICE DELIVERY ISSUES

How then, can one develop an effective service system for the Chinese whose family has such a strong hold on the sick individual? No panacea may be found, but certain measures are suggested in the remaining part of this paper.

It is essential that a mental health service should be physically located in, or close to, the Chinese community to enable it to develop a close and lively relationship of trust with the key leaders and social institutions, e.g., executives of Tang Associations, physicians, pharmacists, herb doctors, schools, churches, culture centres, etc. Once a trust relationship is established, a mental health worker would be able to have contacts with the right people to obtain needed information and support.

Family acceptance of psychiatric intervention for its sick member, especially at an early stage, presents a real challenge to the mental health worker. This can best happen when the family is persuaded about the efficacy of the treatment method to be used. A great deal of patience and understanding of Chinese views on mental illness will be required of the mental health worker to be an effective agent in this regard. Once they are convinced of the "rationality" (You-lee) of the explanation given and of the competence of the worker, their cooperation can be secured.

For the chronic patients who have no family or have been rejected by the family, the multicisciplinary team can be a most effective agent in assisting them to reactivate or rebuild a psychosocial kinship network, (Weiss, 1976).

In the three-year experiences of a mental health team serving Chinese patients in Vancouver, the majority of these chronic patients not only recovered from their psychotic conditions, but also learned social or life skills. They are maintaining a certain level of quality of life among newly found friends in the Chinese community, (Beiser *et al.*, 1978; Bigelow and Beiser, 1978; Goodacre *et al.*, 1975; Nann and Stewart, 1975).

The social and professional status of the mental health worker plays an important role in this process. Physicians or psychiatrists enjoy a special privilege in Chinese society and thus, add a great deal of weight in persuading the patient or the family to accept psychiatric treatment. For a community mental health centre, the presence of a doctor as a member of an interdisciplinary team at its initial contact, and preferably during the first few sessions with the patient and family, is most desirable for maximizing the effect of treatment.

The need for bilingual workers for the Chinese population cannot be overemphasized and consideration should be given to developing a training program of quality. A successful training program presupposes well motivated and intelligent candidates. The small number of Chinese professionals in human services today, due to the traditional lack of interest in community services and also to the typical apathy to mental health in particular, makes the task of recruitment exceedingly difficult. A long term determined effort is needed, which should create more job opportunities to motivate Chinese youth to join in human services.

Language proficiency should not be the sole qualification of a bilingual worker. In addition to professional excellence, deep understanding of culture and the community, familiarity with the key people, and cultural sensitivity to people of various social backgrounds will be required for a bilingual worker to effectively play the role of being a "double agent" — that is, a therapeutic agent and a confidant of the family (Fisher and Miller, 1973; Kadushin, 1972).

Furthermore, they should have an understanding of the traditional concept of mental illness and the ways in which the psychiatric patients are viewed and managed within their families. For such training, practical experience would be most useful in learning the delicate art of approaching the family and the community. A centre of excellence should be established for both service and training. (Murase, 1973).

The use of psychotropic drugs by the Chinese patients deserves a special consideration, both for cultural and technical reasons. Due to their pragmatism, the Chinese tend to test the efficacy of medicines given to them, especially when no full confidence is established between the patient and the therapist. A great deal of care should be given in explaining the medication to the patient and maintaining the effective dosage. One should also keep in mind that the Chinese are constitutionally different from Westerners in terms of sensitivity and tolerance to certain drugs. For example, it is well known that many Chinese or Japanese manic patients respond favourably to lithium carbonate at blood level 0.4 or 0.6, which is lower than that of the Caucasians, and the depressive patients to 50 mg to 75 mg oral doses of amitriptyline, which are considerably smaller in dosages than those for the Caucasians. Such cross-cultural experiences in the use of psychotropic drugs deserve further systematic research.

CONCLUDING REMARKS

In this paper, the author has described and discussed various aspects of sociopsychological and cultural factors in influencing the pattern of help-seeking of Chinese psychiatric patients. Several ideas for developing an effective and relevant mental health service are suggested. How much of the lessons learned from the Chinese are applicable to other Asian groups in North America is a question which can only be answered by further studies. It is our speculation, based on past clinical experiences in Asia and elsewhere, that many of the factors discussed in this paper might have comparable counterparts in some other cultural groups, notably among the Japanese.

In cross-cultural psychiatry, health care delivery issues have been left mostly to administrators and policy-makers who are often not sufficiently sensitive to, nor aware of, the cultural realities of the population at risk (Sue and McKinney, 1975; Hardwick, 1975). Encouragement should be given to research and research training of mental health workers in this field (Giordans, 1973).

REFERENCES

Bancroft, G. (ed.)
    1976 Outreach for understanding, report on intercultural seminars, Chinese. Ontario Ministry of Culture and Recreation, Multicultural Development Branch, Toronto.
Berk, Bernard B. and Hirata, Lucie Cheng
    1973 Mental illness among the Chinese: myth or reality. Journal of Social Issues 19: 149–166.
Beiser, M., Krell, R., Lin, T., Miller, M. (eds.)
    1978 Today's Priorities in Mental Health: Knowing and Doing, Symposia Specialists, Miami, Florida.
Bigelow, Douglas A. and Beiser, Morton
    1978 Rehabilitation for the chronically mentally ill: A community program, Canada's Mental Health 26: 2.
Brody, E. B.
    1970 Migration and adaptation: The nature of the problem, In Behavior in New Environments: Adaptations of Migrant Populations, E. B. Brody (ed.) Sage Publications, Beverly Hills, California.
Chen, Peter W.
    1976 Chinese-Americans view their mental health, DSW dissertation, University of Southern California.
Fisher, Joel and Miller, Henry
    1973 The effect of client race and social class on clinical judgements. Clinical Social Work 1: 100–109.
Fong, S.
    1973 Assimilation and changing social roles of Chinese Americans. Journal of Social Issues 29: 115–128.

Giordans, J.
 1973 Ethnicity and mental health: Research and recommendations. Institute of human relations, New York.
Goodacre, R. H., Coles, E. M., Coates, D. B. et al.
 1975 Hospitalization and hospital bed placement. Canadian Psychiatric Association Journal 20: 00–00.
Hardwick, Frances (ed.)
 1975 East Meets West: A Source Book for the Study of Chinese Immigrants and Their Descendants in Canada. Tentalus Research, Vancouver.
Ho, Man Keung
 1976 Social work with Asian Americans. Social Casework 37: 195–201.
Hsuang, Ken and Pilisuk, Marc
 1977 At the threshold of the Golden Gate: Special problems of a neglected minority. American Journal of Orthopsychiatry 47, (October 4): 00–00.
Ilza, Veith
 1972 The Yellow Emperor's Classic of Internal Medicine. University of California Press, Berkeley.
Kadushin, Alfred
 1972 The racial factor in the interview, Social Work 17: 88–98. Special Issue on 'Enthnicity and Social Work'.
Lin, T., Tardiff, K., Donnetz, G., and Goresky, W.
 1978 Ethnicity and patterns of help-seeking. Culture, Medicine and Psychiatry 2: 3–13.
Lin, Tsung-yi and Lin, Mei-chen
 1978 Service delivery issues in Asian-North American Communities. American Journal of Psychiatry 135: 454–456.
Lyman, S. M., Willmott, W. E., and Ho, B.
 1964 Rules of a Chinese secret society in British Columbia. Bulletin of the School of Oriental and African Studies. University of London, Vol. XXVII, Part 3.
Mead, Margaret
 1970 Culture and Commitment. A Study of the Generation Gap. Natural History Press, New York.
Ministry of Industry, Trade and Commerce
 1971 Statistics Canada, Statistical Information, Vancouver.
Sue, S. and Kitano, H. (eds.)
 1973 Asian American stereotypes as a measure of success. Journal of Social Issues 19: 83–98.
Sue, S. and McKinney, H.
 1975 Asian Americans in the community and mental health care system, American Journal of Orthopsychiatry 45: 111–118.
Thomas, C. and Comer, J.
 1973 Racism and mental health services. In Racism and Mental Health: Essays, C. Willie, B. Kramer and B. Brown (eds.). University of Pittsburgh Press, Pittsburgh.
Weiss, R.
 1976 Transition states and other stressful situations: Their nature and programs for their management. In Support Systems and Mutual Help: Multidisciplinary Explorations, G. Caplan, M. Killilea (eds.). Grunead and Stratton, New York.
Yamamoto, Joe, Quinton, B., Milton, H. Jack
 1967 Racial factors in patient selection, American Journal of Psychiatry 124: 636–637.

LIST OF CONTRIBUTORS

Mary Ashworth, Associate Professor of Language Education, Faculty of Education, University of British Columbia, Vancouver, Canada.
Ali Nahit Babaoglu, M.D., Psychiatrist, Rheinisches Landeskrankenhaus Duren, Duren, West Germany.
Morton Beiser, M.D., Professor of Psychiatry, Faculty of Health Sciences, University of British Columbia, Vancouver, Canada.
Sylvia C. L. Chen, M.B., B.S., MRC (Psych.), Hong Kong Psychiatric Centre, Bonham Road, Hong Kong.
Ben Chud, M.S.W., Associate Professor, School of Social Work, University of British Columbia, Vancouver, Canada.
George V. Coelho, Ph.D., Senior Social Scientist, Office of the Director, National Institute of Mental Health, Rockville, Maryland, U.S.A.
Akira Hoshino, Ph.D., Professor of Psychology, International Christian University, Tokyo, Japan.
K. C. Li, M. B., F.R.C.P. (C.), Psychiatrist, Strathcona Community Care Team, Greater Vancouver Mental Health Service, Vancouver, Canada.
Keh-Ming Lin, M.D., MPH, Department of Psychiatry, Harbor General Hospital, University of California, Los Angeles Medical Center, Torrance, California, U.S.A.
Mei-chen-Lin, Senior Psychiatric School Work Consultant, Strathcona Community Care Team, Greater Vancouver Mental Health Service, Vancouver, Canada.
Norman V. Lourie, M.S.W., D.H.L., Senior Policy Advisor, Institute for Economic Development, Washington, D.C., U.S.A.
Heather Luk, M.A., Strathcona Community Care Team, Greater Vancouver Mental Health Service, Vancouver, Canada.
K. Y. Mak, M.B., B.S., M.R.C.Psych., D.P.M., Hong Kong Psychiatric Centre, Bonham Road, Hong Kong.
Minoru Masuda, Ph.D., Department of Psychiatry and Behavioral Sciences, University of Washington, Seattle, Washington, U.S.A.
Beverly Nann, B.A., B.S.W., Coordinator, The Immigrant Resources Project and the Multicultural Home/School Liaison Project, Vancouver, Canada.
Richard C. Nann, D.S.W., Professor, School of Social Work, University of British Columbia, Vancouver, Canada.
Maria Pfister-Ammende, M.D., President, Schweizerisches Nationalkomitee fur Geistige Gesundheit, Zurich, Switzerland.
Britt-Ingrid Stockfelt-Hoatson, Ph.D., National Immigration and Naturalization Board, Statens Invandrarverk, Sweden.

LIST OF CONTRIBUTORS

Laurie Tazuma, M.D., Neuropsychiatric Institute, Centre For the Health Sciences, University of California, Los Angeles, Westwood, California, U.S.A.

Lilian To, M.S.W., Langley Mental Health Service, Langley, B.C., Canada.

A. L. Th. Verdonk, Ph.D. Department of Preventive and Social Psychiatry, Faculty of Medicine, Erasmus University, Rotterdam, The Netherlands.

Joe Yamamoto, M.D., Neuropsychiatric Institute, Centre For the Health Sciences, University of California, Los Angeles, Westwood, California, U.S.A.

INDEX OF NAMES

Abadan-Unat, N. 118
Abramson, J. H. 23
Adams, J. E. 107
Adams, K. S. 32
Ahmed, P. 107
Alexander, A. A. 101, 107
Alfred, B. M. 119, 139, 143
Almeida, Z. de 64, 68
Alofs, B. 68
Amarasingham, L. 103, 107
Ashworth, Mary 77, 83, 93
Assael, M. 119, 137, 143
Aylesworth, L. S. 138, 143

Babaoglu, Ali Nahit 111
Bagley, C. 68
Bailey, D. E. 146
Bancroft, G. 184
Barger, W. K. 138, 139, 143
Baxter, J. C. 26, 33
Becker, R. 118
Beiser, Morton 119, 125, 126, 132, 140, 143, 183, 184
Benfari, R. C. 143
Bennett, L. 33
Bergman, A. B. 33
Berk, Bernard B. 177, 184
Berkson, D. M. 146
Bernkert, H. 118
Berreman, G. D. 143
Berthelier, R. 68
Bigelow, Douglas A. 183, 184
Boker, W. 118
Bolen, J. S. 21, 23
Bovenkerk, F. 53, 56, 68
Boyce, E. 139, 143
Bramwell, S. T. 26, 32
Brennan, J. 145
Breton, Raymond 93, 155, 163
Brink, P. J. 149, 153
Brislin, R. 107
Brodman, K. 13, 23, 32
Brody, E. B. 67, 139, 143, 184
Brown, A. C. 13, 19, 23
Bruner, E. B. 143
Burgess, E. W. 143
Butcher, J. N. 45, 47

Caplan, G. 66, 68
Carranza, E. 26, 32
Carstairs, G. M. 143
Cawte, J. 143
Celdran, H. H. 26, 32
Chance, N. A. 143
Chen, Peter W. 177, 184
Chen, Sylvia C. L. 147
Chu, H. D. 11, 23
Chu, H. M. 13, 19, 23
Chud, Ben 10. 95
Clark, M. 139, 140, 144
Clinard, J. W. 26, 32
Coates, D. B. 185
Coddington, R. D. 26, 32
Coelho, George V. 101, 105, 106, 107
Coenen, W. 68
Cohen, G. M. 45, 47
Cohen, L. 105, 107
Coles, E. M. 185
Collomb, H. 119, 125, 140, 143
Comer, J. 185
Coplan, A. 104, 105, 107
Cox, J. L. 153
Cutler, D. L. 33

D'Atri, D. A. 145
Davis, A. 67
Davies, R. 32
Delpech, B. 120, 144
Devine, B. 139, 144
De Vos, G. A. 119, 140, 144
Dewson, J. 144
Dohrenwend, B. P. 11, 23, 132, 139, 144
Dohrenwend, B. S. 11, 23, 132, 139, 144
Dollard, J. 67
Donnetz, G. 185

Edwards, A. T. 11, 23
Eisenstadt, S. N. 144
Eitinger, L. 11, 23
Endicott, J. 45, 47
Erdmann, A. J., Jr. 23, 32
Erikson, Erik H. 1, 9, 142, 144
Escudero, M. 145

Fisher, Joel 183, 184

INDEX OF NAMES

Fong, S. 180, 182, 184
Fried, M. 119, 138, 140, 144
Friessem, D. H. 118
Fry, J. 13, 19, 23
Fung, D. 24

Gamble, D. F. 119, 120, 144
Gampel, B. 138, 144
Gans, Herbert J. 155, 163
Geiger, H. J. 138, 146
German, G. A. 119, 143
Giordans, J. 184, 185
Goodacre, R. H. 183, 185
Gordon, J. M. 45, 47
Gordon, T. 139, 144
Goresky, W. 185
Graves, T. D. 119, 139, 144
Griffey, W. P. 143
Grunfeld, B. 11, 23
Guttman, L. 146

Hamburg, D. A. 101, 107
Handlin, O. 67
Harburg, E. 139, 144
Harding, J. S. 145
Hardwick, Frances 184, 185
Harmon, D. K. 26, 32
Hawkins, N. G. 25, 26, 32
Head, Wilson A. 7, 9
Hein, L. 33
Hettinga, N. 60, 68
Hirata, Lucie Cheng 184
Ho, B. 185
Ho, Man Keung 176, 185
Holmes, T. H. 19, 23, 25, 26, 29, 32, 33
Hong, K. E. M. 19, 23
Hoshino, Akira 185
Hsuang, Ken 185
Hughes, C. C. 138, 144, 145
Hunter, J. M. 138, 144
Husain, A. F. A. 138, 144

Iga, M. 24
Ilza, Veith 185
Inkeles, A. 119, 138, 140, 145
Isherwood, J. 26, 32

Janney, J. G. 31, 32
Jacobson, A. 24
Jessor, R. 139, 145

Kabela, M. 64, 69
Kadushin, Alfred 183, 185

Kass, E. H. 145
Kaufman, S. 144
Kessner, T. 67
Kish, L. 124, 145
Kitano, H. H. L. 45, 47, 181, 185
Kjaer, G. 33
Klee, E. 118
Kleiner, R. J. 64, 69, 138, 139, 140
Klineberg, Otto 8, 9, 102, 106, 107
Kok, H. 69
Kramer, Ralph M. 160, 163
Krell, R. 184

Lalonde, M. 102, 107
Lam, J. 24
Lambo, T. A. 145
Lebra, T. S. 46, 47
Lee, Rose Hum 172
Leighton, A. H. 119, 138, 140, 142, 145
Leighton, D. C. 142, 145
Li, K. C. 165
Lin, Keh-Ming 11, 12, 23, 25, 32, 33
Lin, Mei-Chen 172, 175, 177, 181, 185
Lin, Tsung-Yi v, 172, 175, 177, 181, 185
Lin, W. T. 24
Lindberg, H. A. 146
Ling, J. 145
Little, K. 138, 145
Lo, W. H. 153, 154
Loeb, M. B. 24
Looney, J. G. 24
Lourie, Norman V. 35
Luk, Heather 165
Lundeberg, U. 33
Lyman, S. M. 185

McFee, M. 140, 145
McKinney, H. 177, 181, 184, 185
Macklin, D. B. 145
Mak, K. Y. 147
Marris, P. 104, 107
Marsella, A. J. 138, 145
Marzak, R. 57, 69
Masuda, Minoru 11, 13, 19, 23, 25, 26, 29, 32, 33
Mathers, J. 19, 23
Mead, Margaret 9, 182, 185
Meer, Ph. van der 69
Mehrlander, U. 118
Meillasoux, C. 138, 145
Merton, R. 65, 139, 145
Mesman Schultz, K. 69
Meszaros, A. F. 11, 22, 23

INDEX OF NAMES

Methorst, P. 69
Meyer, M. 33
Mezey, A. G. 11, 24
Miall, W. E. 139, 145
Miller, Henry 183, 184
Miller, M. 184
Milton, H. Jack 185
Miner, H. 119, 140, 144
Morrison, S. D. 148, 154
Murase, K. 183
Murphy, H. B. M. 4, 9, 119, 138, 145, 155, 163
Murphy, J. M. 119, 139, 145

Nachman, M. 143
Nakane, C. 46, 47
Nann, Beverly 85, 93
Nann, Richard C. 1, 9, 10, 155, 163, 173, 183
Needelman, B. 69
Ness, R. 145

Oaski, L. T. 143
Odegaard, O. 11, 24
O'Donnell, Edward J. 160, 163
Ossario, P. G. 143
Ostfeld, A. M. 145

Padilla, E. R. 26, 33
Panchari, P. 47
Park, R. 65, 69
Parker, S. 64, 69, 138, 139, 140, 145
Pedersen, P. B. 105, 107
Pederson, S. 11, 24
Pfister-Ammende, M. xiii, xv, 118
Pierce, R. C. 144
Pilisuk, Marc 185
Polgar, S. 137, 145

Quinton, B. 185

Rahe, R. H. 20, 24, 25, 26, 31, 33
Ravel, J. L. 143
Remy, M. 122, 145
Reverdy, J. C. 120, 122, 145
Rin, H. 13, 19, 23
Rockwell, B. 69
Rohsenow, D. J. 33
Ruesch, R. D. 21, 24
Rumbaut, R. D. 11, 20, 24
Rumbaut, R. G. 11, 20, 24

Saran, P. 105, 107

Saunders, J. M. 149, 153
Scotch, N. A. 119, 138, 146
Seebaran, R. 7, 10
Selzer, M. L. 26, 33
Senghor, L. S. 119, 146
Seppa, M. T. 26, 33
Slome, C. 144
Slotkin, J. S. 146
Smedes, D. H. 119, 138, 140, 145
Smith, M. 33
Soetens, N. 58, 69
Spanje, N. C. B. 69
Spaulding, S. 105, 106, 107
Spitzer, R. L. 45, 47
Stamler, J. 139, 146
Stein, J. J. 101, 107
Stevens, S. S. 33
Stewart, P. 163, 183
Stockfelt-Hoatson, B.-I. 71
Stouffer, S. A. 128, 146
Strauch, P. 144
Strong, E. K. 67
Suchman, E. A. 146
Sue, S. 177, 181, 184, 185
Sullivan, Marilyn M. 160, 163

Tan, F. 24
Tardiff, K. 185
Tazuma, Laurie 11, 25, 33
Theorell, T. 33
Thomas, C. 185
To, Lilian 155
Triandis, H. 105, 107
Tryon, R. C. 124, 146
Tung, T. M. 24
Turner, R. H. 146
Tyhurst, L. 11, 22, 24

Valdes, T. M. 26, 33
Verdonk, A. L. Th. 49, 52, 54, 56, 64, 65, 70
Verveen-Keulemans, F. M. 70
Vinokur, A. 26, 33

Wagner, N. 32, 33
Ward, H. W. 24
Weiss, R. 182, 185
White, R. H. 101, 107
Wierx, R. 69
Willmott, William E. 155, 163, 185
Wirth, Louis 155, 163
Wolff, H. G. 23, 32
Woon, T. 26, 33

Wyler, A. R. 26, 33

Yamamoto, J. 21, 24, 41, 185

Zwingmann, C. A. 118

INDEX OF SUBJECTS

Affiliated Asian-American Mental Health Task Force 41
aggressive attitudes in refugees 22
Asian-American Mental Health Training Center 41

bilingualism and biculturalism 71-75, 88

California Agencies working with Indo-Chinese refugees 38
children of foreign workers in the Netherlands 53-56, 61
children of immigrants
   in Canada 77-81, 91
   in the Netherlands 49-50
   in Sweden 71-72
Chinese culture and the adjustment problems of immigration 171
Chinese immigrants in Canada 155-156
   case histories of patients 166-171
   mental health services for 165-166
   patterns of help-seeking 176
   socio-economic status 156-157
Chinese in Taiwan 19
Chinese-speaking Vietnamese 21
common settlement experiences of immigrants 86
Cornell Medical Index (CMI) 12, 25
culture shock 86, 101-102, 104, 109

depressive problems among refugees 22
discrimination and intolerance 87

economic adaptation 5, 50-51, 54-55, 87, 112, 120
education and language training of immigrant children and their families 81
   (*see also*: ESL and schooling)
educational adaptation 6, 80, 82
ESL classes (English as a Second Language) 77-78, 81
   bilingual "head start" instruction 91
   training for ESL teachers 82
ethnic community 3, 138
ethnic support system
   philosophy and objectives 158

programs and services 158-160
foreign students 101-108
foreign workers 53-58, 111-118

generational communication gap 88
Greater Vancouver Mental Health Service 165

identity crisis among immigrant children xv, 5, 60, 73, 88
immigrant wives and mothers
   parenting dilemmas 87
   special needs of 5, 85
immigration and refugee settlement in Canada 156
Indian students in the United States 103
indigenous ethnic institutions as sources of social support 155
International Christian University in Tokyo 110
International Year of the Child xii

Japanese culture and Japanese-Americans 45
   patterns of behavior and implications for therapy 46
Japanese youth 109-110

Korean Mental Health Center in Los Angeles 44

language and cultural roots of migrant populations 3, 72
language needs and staffing of services 41-42, 91, 183
life changes among Vietnamese refugees 25, 28-29

mainland Chinese in Hong Kong 147-148
   mental health aspects 151-152
mental health service delivery issues 182-184
mental health services in Hong Kong 148
migration in a developing country 119-120

INDEX OF SUBJECTS

Moluccans in the Netherlands 50-51, 59

New Orleans Associated Catholic Charities 38

Pennsylvania Office of Mental Health 40
planning and delivery of resettlement services 6-8, 35-40, 41-44, 88-89, 105, 160-162, 182-183
post-war immigrants to Canada 77
program outcomes and limitations 160
psychiatric status schedule 45

racist and sexist stereotyping in textbooks 82
religion and cultural transition 15, 73
Rheinisches Landeskrankenhaus Duren 113
rural-urban migration and adjustment 86, 119-120, 132-136

Salzburg Congress xii
Schedule of Recent Experience (SRE) 12, 26
school-based service programs for immigrant families and children 7, 89, 105
schooling of immigrant children
 adapting to a new system 88
 deviant behavior patterns 78-79
 emotional problems and linguistic inadequacy 75
 home influences 79-80
 teachers and immigrant students 74-75
Serer of Senegal 120-122
 health and mental health data 129-132
 living in Dakar 125
Social Readjustment Rating Questionnaire (SRRQ) 12, 25-26
 cross cultural studies 29
 status inconsistency 21, 87

Strathcona Community Care Team 165
Surinamese and Antillians in the Netherlands 51-53, 59-60

theories about psychological problems 63-64
traditional Chinese view on mental illness 177
 etiology of mental illness 179
 family response to and intervention in mental health problems 180-181
 social stigma and shame 177
 Yin and Yang: imbalance of, and mental illness 179
Turkish workers in West Germany
 demographic characteristics 111-113
 life goals 113
 psychiatric aspects 113-117
two typologies of adaptation 139-140
types of migration and mobility xv

University of Dakar Medical School 126
University of Washington Department of Psychiatry and Behavioral Sciences 12
uprooting 1-2, 11, 35, 104
 "double" uprooting 101, 109
 measures for prevention xv, 66
 physical 86
 psychological 86

Vancouver Congress xii
Vienna Congress xiii
Vietnamese refugees in the United States 11-24, 25-34
village cooperative movement of Senegal 120

Wisconsin Resettlement Assistance Office 37